CURRENT CLINICAL NEUROLOGY

Daniel Tarsy, MD, SERIES EDITOR

Roongroj Bhidayasiri • Daniel Tarsy

Movement Disorders:
A Video Atlas

☼ Humana Press

Roongroj Bhidayasiri, MD, FRCP, FRCPI
Chulalongkorn Center of Excellence on
Parkinson's Disease and Related Disorders
Chulalongkorn University Hospital
Bangkok
Thailand

Department of Neurology
David Geffen School of Medicine at UCLA
Los Angeles, CA
USA

Daniel Tarsy, MD
Department of Neurology
Harvard Medical School
Beth Israel Deaconess Medical Center
Boston, MA
USA

ISBN 978-1-60327-425-8   ISBN 978-1-60327-426-5   (eBook)
DOI 10.1007/978-1-60327-426-5
Springer New York Heidelberg Dordrecht London

Library of Congress Control Number: 2012941848

Printed on acid-free paper

Humana Press is a brand of Springer
Springer is part of Springer Science+Business Media (www.springer.com)

To my beloved grandmother Pranom Chivakiat, my parents Mitr and Nisaratana Bhidayasiri, and all my teachers of neurology who have taught me so much about neurology and movement disorders.

Roongroj Bhidayasiri, MD, FRCP, FRCPI

To Professor C. David Marsden who continues to be an inspiration in my life, and to my beloved wife who has always loved, understood, and supported me.

Daniel Tarsy, MD

Foreword

There is a statement by Sir William Osler in his remarks at the 1901 dedication ceremony for a new building of the Boston Medical Library that can be aptly applied to this volume by Drs. Bhidayasiri and Tarsy. Osler said, "To study the phenomenon of disease without books is to sail an uncharted sea, while to study books without patients is not to go to sea at all." Similarly, with the wide variety of phenomenologies of movement disorders – we need to witness them in order to identify, classify, and treat them. Reading about movement disorders is insufficient. Words cannot adequately describe the various abnormal movements encountered in patients who have developed certain neurological conditions, now uniformly called movement disorders. Only seeing them can make one's mind recognize them. Witnessing the abnormal movements via cinematography or videotapes is the next best thing to examining the live patient. The reader, or should I say viewer, of this treatise will have the benefit of Drs. Bhidayasiri and Tarsy's efforts. And effort it is. As a movement disorder specialist who takes videotapes of patients, I can appreciate the work involved in selecting the ideal cases and editing the tapes to a reasonable length that allows the viewer to obtain the essential observations without extraneous material that would make the video segment boring.

Cinematography of movement disorders began when the movie camera was available to the public. The commercial 16-mm film was standard, and, of course, the movies were silent in those early days. Some neurologists took advantage of this new technology and made movies during the 1920s and 1930s of the cases of postencephalitic parkinsonism and hyperkinesias that occurred following the pandemics of encephalitis lethargic. The technique was also used to record many other movement disorders. When sound became available, professional-type movies were created for teaching medical students about neurological conditions. I recall seeing a film on abnormal gaits when I was a resident in neurology.

When 8-mm home movie cameras became available, these were adopted by some neurologists, including myself, who would "shoot" their patients. These films, with editing, were utilized at courses, including the movement disorder courses and the Unusual Movement Disorder seminars at the annual meetings of the American Academy of Neurology, beginning in 1981. Technology has advanced, and cinematography gave way to videotaping. Videos had many advantages over film – instantaneous access without developing the film, viewing without an elaborate setup, and especially the incorporation of sound. As video cameras became smaller, a movement disorder neurologist not only has it readily available in the office setting but is also able to carry the camera with him on rounds, as he would a reflex hammer, and be ready to "shoot" a patient with abnormal movements who might be on the wards. Videotapes of movement disorders shown at neurology meetings have set the standards in unifying how abnormal movements are classified.

Not only do neurologists need to know how to diagnose the abnormal movements but so should other physicians and other medical personnel, such as nurses, physiotherapists, and occupational therapists. Having a reference source, such as this Video Atlas, is a welcome addition in the education of neurologists and other medical personnel on the variety of movement disorders. We all appreciate the work and dedication that Drs. Bhidayasiri and Tarsy exerted to bring us this useful educational treatise.

Stanley Fahn, MD
H. Houston Merritt Professor of Neurology
Director, Center for Parkinson's Disease
and Other Movement Disorders
Columbia University
New York, NY
USA

Preface

The use of video has been a vital tool for the display of clinical phenomenology in patients with movement disorders for at least the past 40 years. Those of us in the field are indebted to Dr. Stanley Fahn who introduced and promoted its use, first in his own department at Columbia University, and later in national and international meetings of the Movement Disorders Society and other neurological organizations. For example, the Unusual Movement Disorders Course presented at the annual meeting of the American Academy of Neurology has been a popular mainstay of video demonstration and teaching for several decades. In 1986, as the first editors of the journal *Movement Disorders*, Dr. Fahn and Professor C. David Marsden introduced video supplements in the form of VHS videotape to illustrate cases described in selected articles and case reports in the journal. This first use of video journal supplements became an instant hit with the readership of the *Movement Disorders* journal and, with changes in available technology, has advanced over the years to DVD-ROMs and finally to online access of video material.

Following Dr. Fahn's lead, regular movement disorders videoconferences became widespread in neurology departments in the United States and around the world. Video has also become extensively used for teaching purposes on the Movement Disorders Society website, at local, national, and international movement disorders meetings and courses, and is commonly circulated by email among colleagues for informal consultation concerning unusual cases. The use of patient video has since caught on in many other clinical specialties. Several medical journals now provide online video supplements, and video presentations are commonly used at clinical meetings and courses in many medical specialties.

In this video atlas, we have put together a series of cases representing patients with parkinsonism, tremor, dystonia, chorea, myoclonus, cerebellar ataxia, and tic disorders.

For each case, we have provided background, a brief case report, and a description of the video. For purchasers of this book, the videos are available at the Springer website www.springerimages.com/Tarsy, where they can be viewed while referring to the source material provided in this volume. Some are narrated while others retain original audio of the physician-patient interchange. We are hopeful that this case collection will continue to grow as we add additional cases and video online. We greatly appreciate the help and support of Richard Lansing at Humana Press/ Springer who helped to make this work a reality. We are also grateful for the tireless work of Tom Laws and the Media Services department of Beth Israel Deaconess Medical Center for their assistance in this project. Finally, we are very indebted to our patients and their families whose continued courage and cooperation in the face of great personal adversity have contributed to our own education and the education of movement disorder doctors around the world.

Roongroj Bhidayasiri, MD, FRCP, FRCPI
Daniel Tarsy, MD

Contents

Part IV: Choreiform Disorders

Part V: Myoclonus

Part VI: Cerebellar Ataxia

Contributors

We would like to thank the following contributors who kindly provided us with their very interesting video clips to add to our own collections.

Parnsiri Chairangsaris, M.D. Division of Neurology, Pramongkutklao Hospital, Bangkok, Thailand

Antonio V. Delgado-Escueta, M.D., Ph.D. Department of Neurology, UCLA School of Medicine, Los Angeles, CA, USA

Priya Jagota, M.D. Chulalongkorn Center of Excellence on Parkinson's Disease and Related Disorders, Chulalongkorn University Hospital, Bangkok, Thailand

Asha Kishore, M.D. Sree Chitra Tirunal Institute for Medical Sciences and Technology, Trivandrum, Kerala, India

Kongkiat Kulkantrakorn, M.D. Division of Neurology, Thammasat University Hospital, Pathumthani, Thailand

Helen Ling, M.D., M.Sc. Division of Neurology, Chiang-Mai University Hospital, Chiang-Mai, Thailand

Susan L. Perlman, M.D. Department of Neurology, UCLA School of Medicine, Los Angeles, CA, USA

Yoshikuni Mizuno, M.D., Ph.D. Department of Neurology, Juntendo University School of Medicine, Tokyo, Japan

Kammant Phanthumchinda, M.D., M.Sc. Chulalongkorn Center of Excellence on Parkinson's Disease and Related Disorders, Chulalongkorn University Hospital, Bangkok, Thailand

Nutan Sharma, M.D. Department of Neurology, Massachusetts General Hospital, Boston, MA, USA

Ludy Shih, M.D. Department of Neurology, Beth Israel Deaconess Medical Center, Boston, MA, USA

Part I
Parkinsonism and Related Disorders

Chapter 1
Examination of a Patient with Parkinson's Disease

This chapter contains a video segment which can be found at the
URL: http://www.springerimages.com/Tarsy

Background

Parkinson's disease (PD) is associated with a combination of characteristic clinical
signs which usually allow for prompt and accurate diagnosis. The three cardinal signs
of parkinsonism are tremor, rigidity, and bradykinesia. The presence of at least two of
these signs is required for the diagnosis of PD. Postural instability is a fourth clinical
sign but less useful for early diagnosis as it typically appears later in the course of PD
and is a common feature of other forms of parkinsonism. Although the diagnosis of
parkinsonism can also be made by dopamine reuptake brain imaging, it is not neces-
sary in the majority of cases as long as a careful and critical neurological examination
is carried out by an experienced examiner. The motor portion of the Unified Parkinson's
Disease Rating Scale (UPDRS) forms the basis of the motor examination of the patient
with PD, most of which is illustrated in the accompanying video.

Case

A 65-year-old woman presented with resting tremor in her right hand together with
right shoulder pain. Initial examination showed low amplitude resting tremor in
right hand, mild rigidity in the wrists and in cervical muscles, bilaterally reduced
arm swing, and no other motor findings. Over the next 1–2 years, tremor became
more persistent and she developed increasing and more intrusive bradykinesia in
her right hand. Treatment with pramipexole followed by levodopa/carbidopa
improved her bradykinesia while the tremor remained unchanged.

References

1. Tarsy D. Initial treatment of Parkinson's disease. Curr Treat Options Neurol. 2006;8:224–35.
2. Goetz CG, Stebbins GT, Chmura TA, et al. Teaching tape for the motor section of unified
   Parkinson's Disease rating scale. Mov Disord. 1995;10:263–6.
3. Goetz CG, Tilley BC, Shaftman SR, et al. Movement Disorder Society-sponsored revision of
   the Unified Parkinson's Disease Rating Scale (MDS-UPDRS): scale presentation and clinimet-
   ric testing results. Mov Disord. 2008;23:2129–70.

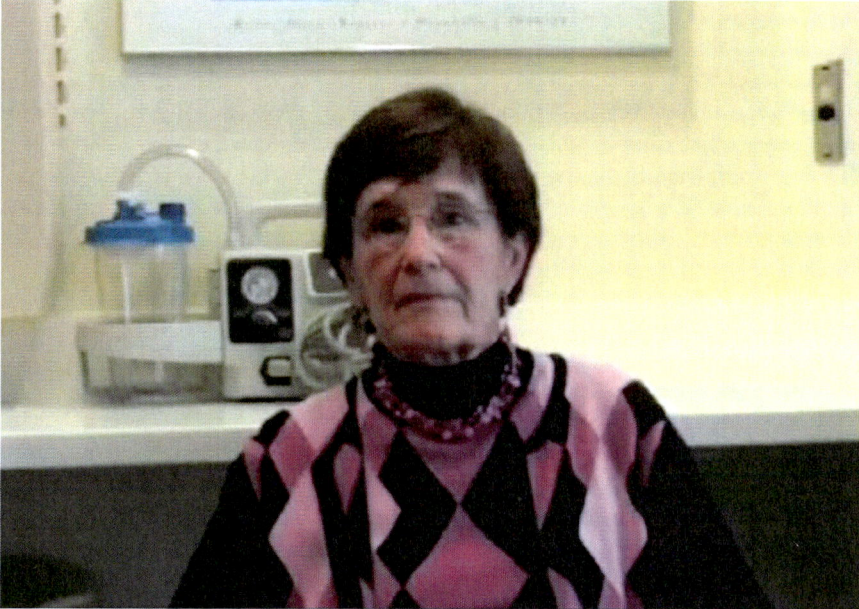

Video
The patient is examined using elements of the motor portion of the UPDRS. There is obvious facial masking and a quiet, monotonic voice. Her arms are folded in her lap with a flexed posture at the metacarpal-phalangeal joints. There is bilateral resting tremor in her hands which increases while reciting months of the year backward. With arms extended, there is a milder, intermittent postural tremor of her hands. Bradykinesia is tested with rapid alternating movements. Rapid finger tapping is quick bilaterally but with small amplitude movements. Rapid wrist rotations and toe tapping movements are associated with a decremental response over several seconds. Rapid open-close hand movements and heel tapping are close to normal. She is able to stand up easily without use of hands. Gait is quick but with markedly reduced arm swing, mildly stooped posture, en bloc turns without extra steps, and activated hand tremor bilaterally. Pull test (not shown) was negative.

Chapter 2
Parkinson's Disease: Hoehn and Yahr Scale

This chapter contains a video segment which can be found at the
URL: http://www.springerimages.com/Tarsy

Background

The Hoehn and Yahr scale (HY) is a widely used clinical rating scale, which defines broad categories of motor function in Parkinson's disease (PD). Among its advantages are that it is simple and easily applied. It captures typical patterns of progressive motor impairment which can be applied whether or not patients are receiving dopaminergic therapy. Progression in HY stages has been found to correlate with motor decline, deterioration in quality of life, and neuroimaging studies of dopaminergic loss. However, because of its simplicity and lack of detail, the scale is not comprehensive. It is also limited by its focus on issues of unilateral versus bilateral disease and the presence or absence of postural reflex impairment, thereby leaving other specific aspects of motor deficit unassessed. Also it does not provide any information concerning nonmotor aspects of PD. A modified version of HY is sometimes used.

Hoehn and Yahr Scale	Modified Hoehn and Yahr Scale
1: Only unilateral involvement, usually with minimal or no functional disability	1.0: Unilateral involvement only
	1.5: Unilateral and axial involvement
2: Bilateral or midline involvement without impairment of balance	2.0: Bilateral involvement without impairment of balance
3: Bilateral disease: mild to moderate disability with impaired postural reflexes; physically independent	2.5: Mild bilateral disease with recovery on pull test
	3.0: Mild to moderate bilateral disease; some postural instability; physically independent
4: Severely disabling disease; still able to walk or stand unassisted	4.0: Severe disability; still able to walk or stand unassisted
5: Confinement to bed or wheelchair unless aided	5.0: Wheelchair bound or bedridden unless aided

References

1. Hoehn MM, Yahr MD. Parkinsonism: onset, progression, and mortality. Neurology. 1967; 17:427–42.
2. Goetz CG, Poewe W, Rascol O, et al. Movement disorder society task force report on the Hoehn and Yahr staging scale: status and recommendations. Mov Disord. 2004;19:1020–8.

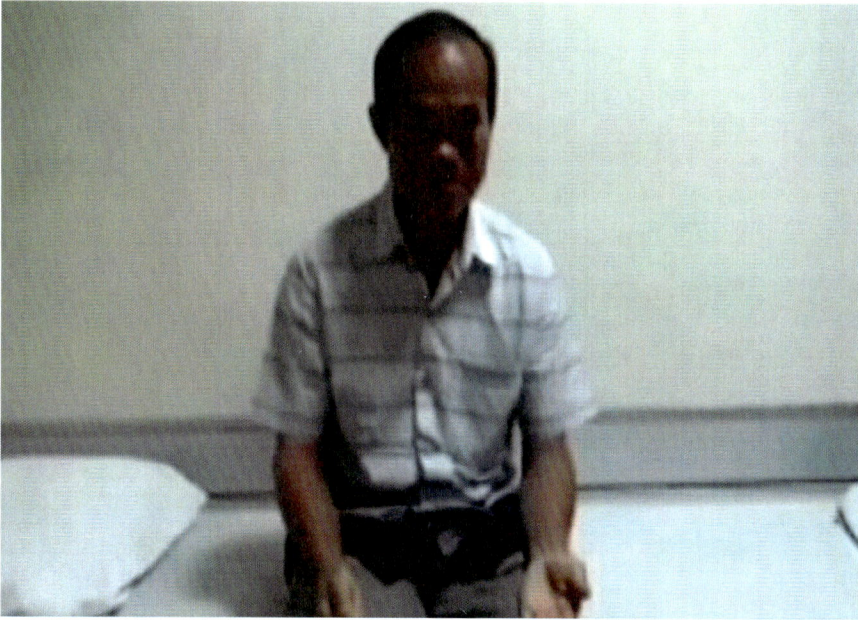

Video

There are five video clips which illustrate patients at HY stages 1–5.

Clip 1: HY1. The patient exhibits resting tremor in right hand and impaired rapid wrist rotations in right wrist. Facial expression appears normal. Gait is brisk and right arm swing is reduced in amplitude but present bilaterally. Clip 2: HY2. The patient exhibits continuous large amplitude resting tremor in both upper extremities, which persists as an action tremor during finger-nose-finger testing. There is prominent facial masking. Gait and turns are normal but with reduced arm swing bilaterally. Hand tremor activates while walking. Rapid alternating movements are slow in both upper extremities. Pull testing (not shown) is normal. Clip 3: HY3. Tremor is absent and facial expression is mildly reduced. Rapid open-close hand movements and wrist rotations are normal but rapid finger tapping is slow in right hand. There appears to be rigidity to passive manipulation in both upper extremities. The patient arises easily without use of hands. Gait is brisk with good arm swing, but while turning the patient displays freezing of gait and gait ignition failure. Pull testing is repeatedly positive. Clip 4: HY4. Facial masking is prominent. There is bilateral resting and postural tremor in upper extremities. The patient requires assistance to stand. The patient is able to walk independently with flexed posture, absent arm swing, shortened stride length, and activated hand tremor. Clip 5: HY5. The patient is wheelchair bound and flexed at waist. There is global akinesia with very slow and poorly maintained rapid alternating hand movements. The patient requires assistance to stand and must be led in order to walk with persistent flexed posture and shortened stride length.

Chapter 3
Young-Onset Parkinson's Disease

This chapter contains a video segment which can be found at the
URL: http://www.springerimages.com/Tarsy

Background

Young-onset Parkinson's disease (YOPD) is arbitrarily defined as Parkinson's disease which produces initial symptoms between ages 21 and 39. YOPD appears to be the same nosologic entity as older-onset Parkinson's disease (PD). It accounts for approximately 5% of PD referrals in Western countries and about 10% in Japan. Compared with older-onset PD, the available evidence suggests that YOPD patients have (1) slower disease progression, (2) an increased frequency of dystonia at onset and during treatment, (3) a lower occurrence of dementia, and (4) an increased risk of dyskinesias in response to levodopa treatment. YOPD appears to form a heterogeneous patient group with a higher proportion of cases due to genetic causes. Approximately 9–20% of patients with YOPD have mutations in the parkin gene, with an additional 1% of cases related to mutations in the *PINK1* and *DJ1* genes.

Case

A 38-year-old man presented with a 2-year history of left arm stiffness. He was initially diagnosed with left shoulder tendonitis and treated unsuccessfully with nonsteroidal anti-inflammatory agents and physical therapy. Recently his colleagues noticed he was limping and appeared to have reduced strength in his left leg. Examination revealed marked bradykinesia in his left hand together with moderate rigidity of his left arm and leg. Tremor was absent. Left arm swing was reduced and there was slight focal dystonia. Handwriting was micrographic. Slit lamp examination showed no Kayser-Fleischer rings and ceruloplasmin level was normal.

References

1. Golbe LI. Young-onset Parkinson's disease: a clinical review. Neurology. 1991;41:168–73.
2. Quinn N, Critchley P, Marsden CD. Young onset Parkinson's disease. Mov Disord. 1987; 2:73–91.
3. Wickremaratchi MM, Ben-Shlomo Y, Morris HR. The effect of onset age on the clinical features of Parkinson's disease. Eur J Neurol. 2009;16:450–6.

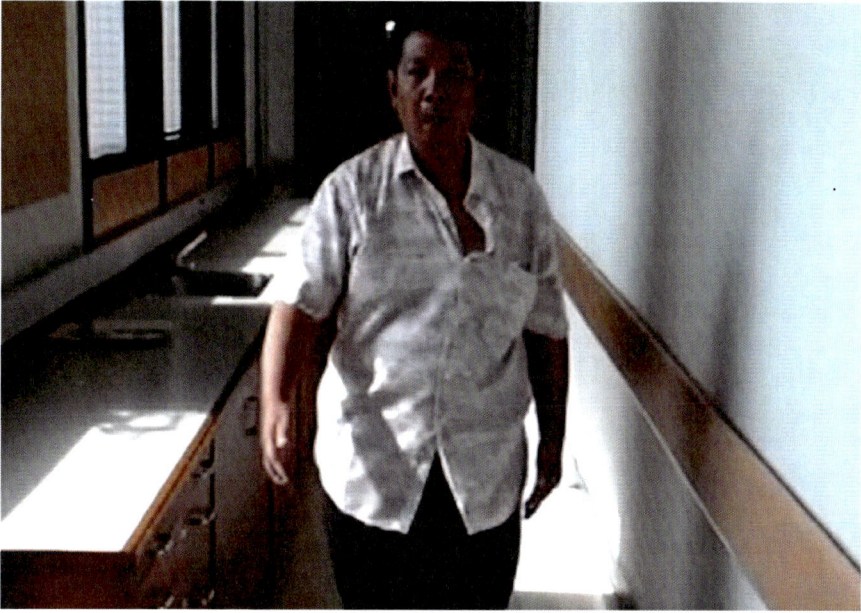

Video
Gait and turns are normal but left arm swing is reduced. There is facial masking. Left-sided rapid hand movements and finger tapping are markedly bradykinetic.

Chapter 4
Tremor-Dominant Parkinson's Disease

This chapter contains a video segment which can be found at the
URL: http://www.springerimages.com/Tarsy

Background

Tremor-dominant Parkinson's disease (PD) refers to patients who present initially
with tremor with relatively mild bradykinesia and rigidity and who progress slowly
over many years with tremor remaining the most prominent clinical symptom together
with relatively mild bradykinesia, rigidity, and absence of postural instability. Several
reports have subtyped patients with PD in order to compare their projected course
over time. In PD, the disease process continues throughout life in a nonlinear fashion
without spontaneous or treatment-induced remission. Although different subtyping
schemes have been proposed, the most well-defined groups to emerge have been the
tremor dominant, akinetic-rigid, and postural instability-gait disturbance (PIGD) subtypes. Longitudinal studies have shown that age of onset is younger and progression
to Hoehn and Yahr stage 4 is slower in tremor-dominant cases. Dementia is more
likely to occur and to be more severe in akinetic-rigid cases and to be less common in
tremor-dominant patients. The annual rates of motor decline as measured by the
Unified Parkinson's Disease Rating Scale, adjusted for age at the initial visit, were
steeper for the PIGD group than for the tremor-dominant group.

Case

A 64-year-old woman with PD presented with resting tremor of the left hand which
was present for 5 years. Although she found that medications were only partially
effective in reducing tremor, she denied symptoms of bradykinesia or gait difficulty.
She was also having no levodopa related motor complications. Examination revealed
left hand resting tremor with only mild bradykinesia and rigidity.

References

1. Jankovic J, Kapadia AS. Functional decline in Parkinson disease. Arch Neurol. 2001;
   58:1611–5.
2. Rajput AH, Sitte H, Rajput A, et al. Globus pallidus dopamine and Parkinson motor subtypes:
   clinical and brain biochemical correlation. Neurology. 2008;70:1403–10.
3. Rajput AH, Voll A, Rajput ML, et al. Course in Parkinson disease subtypes. A 39-year clinico-
   pathologic study. Neurology. 2009;73:206–12.

R. Bhidayasiri, D. Tarsy, *Movement Disorders: A Video Atlas*, Current Clinical Neurology,
DOI 10.1007/978-1-60327-426-5_4, © Springer Science+Business Media New York 2012

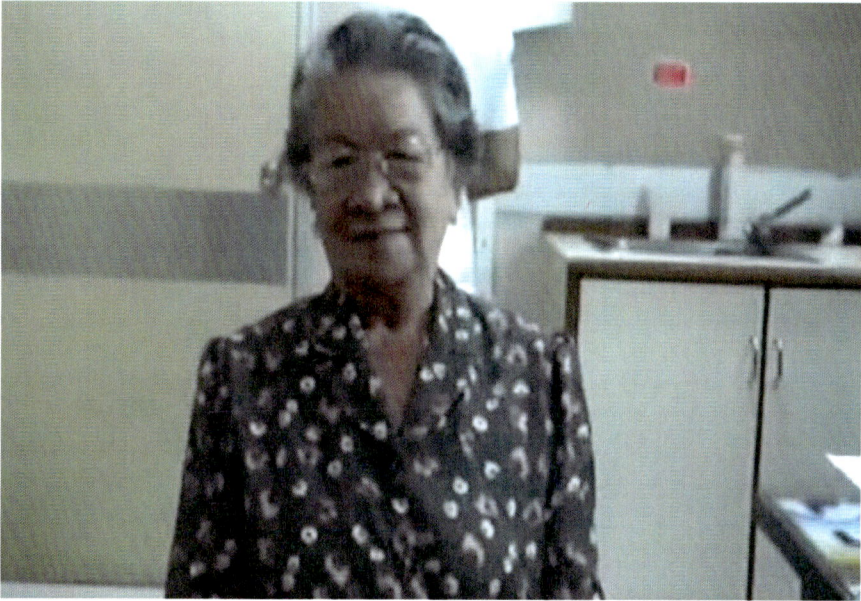

Video

The patient exhibits a large amplitude left hand resting tremor with re-emergent tremor of the left arm after several seconds when her arms are elevated. Facial expression is normal.

Chapter 5
Parkinson's Disease: Levodopa-Induced Dyskinesia

This chapter contains a video segment which can be found at the
URL: http://www.springerimages.com/Tarsy

Background

Although very effective, chronic levodopa therapy for Parkinson's disease (PD) is frequently complicated by the subsequent development of motor complications, which take the form of fluctuations of bradykinesia, rigidity, and tremor- and levodopa-induced dyskinesia and dystonia. With each year of levodopa treatment, about 10% of patients develop motor complications. Young age of PD onset, disease duration and severity, and high doses of levodopa are recognized risk factors for the appearance of motor complications. These complications continue to be a source of disability for PD patients and are a major limiting factor in the therapeutic efficacy of levodopa.

Several types of dyskinesias exist. The most common is peak-dose dyskinesia, which occurs when levodopa's effects on parkinsonism reach their peak effect about 30–90 min after a dose. Peak-dose dyskinesia is usually choreoathetotic, often begins in the foot on the side most affected by PD, and later variably spreads to involve other extremities, the trunk, and facial muscles. In some cases, dyskinesias may be dystonic or ballistic in character. When more severe, dyskinesias may persist throughout most of the "on" period during which time patients may be experiencing adequate motor function. The second type, diphasic dyskinesia ("dyskinesia-improvement-dyskinesia"), is dyskinesia that appears at the beginning of the "on" period, subsides spontaneously, and reappears again as the levodopa effect begins to wear off. End-of-dose dyskinesias come on abruptly with repetitive kicking or bicycling movements of the lower limbs and are often associated with parkinsonian features in the upper half of the body. The third type of dyskinesia is painful off-period dystonia that frequently involves the foot and toes and occurs when parkinsonism becomes apparent. This may occur as some or all doses wear off but sometimes appears only in the early morning when patients have been without levodopa overnight.

Case

A 65-year-old woman with an 8-year history of PD presented with involuntary movements between doses of levodopa. The movements became more severe since her levodopa doses had been increased 2 months previously and were now affecting the entire body. During episodes, which usually lasted for 1–2 h, she could not stand, walk, or perform her daily activities. Examination revealed choreiform movements

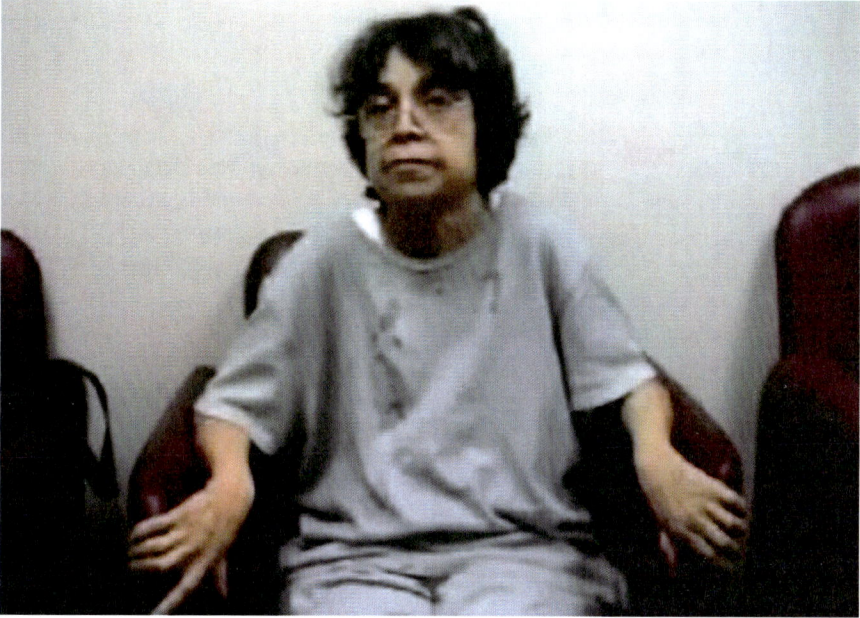

Video
The patient shows choreiform movements involving the entire body, more prominently in the legs, hands, trunk, and neck. She could not suppress these movements. Examination revealed impaired balance together with cervical and upper extremity dyskinesia and dystonic posturing. Tremor and rigidity are minimal during the period of dyskinesia.

affecting all four extremities, associated with body, head, and neck sway to either side. Only minimal rigidity was observed while dyskinesia was present. However, left hand tremor and bradykinesia returned 1 h before her next dose of levodopa.

References

1. Bhidayasiri R, Truong DD. Motor complications in Parkinson disease: clinical manifestations and management. J Neurol Sci. 2008;266:204–15.
2. Calabresi P, Di Filippo M, Ghiglieri V, et al. Levodopa-induced dyskinesias in patients with Parkinson's disease: filling the bench-to-bedside gap. Lancet Neurol. 2010;9:1106–17.
3. Nutt JG. Levodopa-induced dyskinesia: review, observations, and speculations. Neurology. 1990;40:340–5.

Chapter 6
Parkinson's Disease: Diphasic Dyskinesia

This chapter contains a video segment which can be found at the
URL: http://www.springerimages.com/Tarsy

Background

Diphasic dyskinesia (DD) is a complex pattern of levodopa (LD) dyskinesia in patients
with Parkinson's disease (PD) in which involuntary movements occur during both
peak and trough LD effects. End of dose dyskinesia is usually more severe and often
differs in appearance from peak-dose dyskinesia. It commonly causes ballistic flexion-
extension, kicking, or bicycling leg movements which often force the patient into a
reclining position. There may be associated dystonic postures, mental distress, and
autonomic manifestations. DD often occurs toward the end of the day and may sometimes occur only once daily following the final dose of LD when it has been called
"evening dyskinesia." DD is difficult to manage. The use of high-frequency LD doses
and the addition of dopamine agonists or catechol-o-methyl transferase (COMT)
inhibitors to avoid trough effects are only sometimes helpful. To be prevented, end of
day or evening dyskinesia may require high-frequency LD administration around the
clock which is impractical and may cause other LD-related adverse effects. Deep
brain stimulation has occasionally been used successfully for management of DD.

Case

A 64-year-old woman with an 11-year history of PD required LD every 2 h while
working between 8 a.m. and 2 p.m. Once daily, beginning 2 h after her last dose of
LD at 2 p.m., she developed painful dystonia in her right foot followed immediately
by ballistic dyskinesias involving both legs associated with emotional distress and
hyperventilation. Increasing LD dose intervals to 2.5 h resulted in similar end of
dose dyskinesia appearing 2 h following each dose with no change in the end of day
dyskinesias. Lowering of LD dose and addition of sustained release LD, pramipexole, entacapone, and amantadine were all unhelpful. Bilateral subthalamic nucleus
deep brain stimulation (DBS) was carried out. Following DBS programming, LD
was discontinued and pramipexole was reintroduced with resolution of end of day
dyskinesia which was sustained for the next 18 months. LD was reintroduced
8 months after DBS to manage mild LD wearing off effects with appearance of mild
peak dose dyskinesia but without reappearance of end of day dyskinesia.

R. Bhidayasiri, D. Tarsy, *Movement Disorders: A Video Atlas*, Current Clinical Neurology,
DOI 10.1007/978-1-60327-426-5_6, © Springer Science+Business Media New York 2012

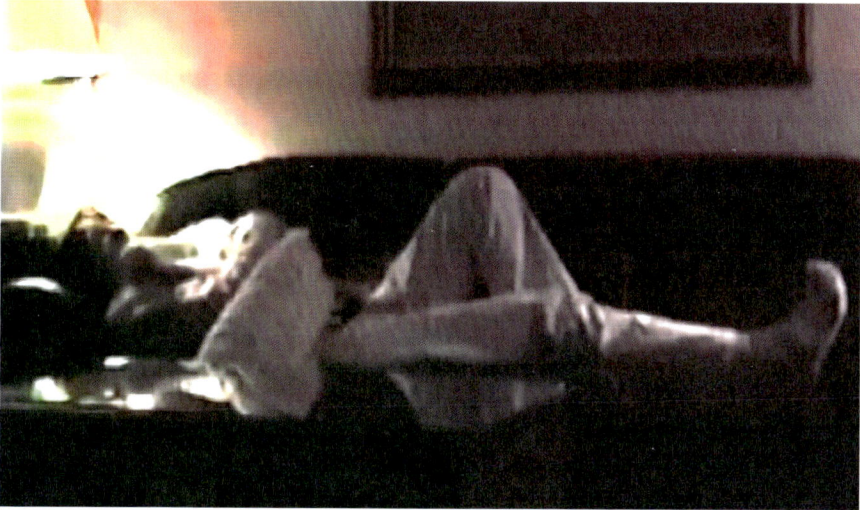

Video
The patient is reclining on a couch with continuous jerky dystonic posturing in her upper limbs and trunk and repetitive kicking movements of the right leg.

References

1. Apetauerova D, Ryan R, Ro SI, et al. End of day dyskinesia in advanced Parkinson's disease can be eliminated by bilateral STN or GPi deep brain stimulation. Mov Disord. 2006;21:1277–9.
2. Zimmerman TR, Sage JL, Lang AE, Mark MH. Severe evening dyskinesias in advanced Parkinson's disease: clinical description, relation to plasma levodopa, and treatment. Mov Disord. 1994;9:173–7.

Chapter 7
Parkinson's Disease: "On-Off" Phenomenon

This chapter contains a video segment which can be found at the
URL: http://www.springerimages.com/Tarsy

Background

The "on-off" phenomenon in Parkinson's disease (PD) refers to a switch between
mobility and immobility in levodopa-treated patients, which occurs as an end-of-
dose or "wearing off" worsening of motor function or, much less commonly, as
sudden and unpredictable motor fluctuations. Motor complications occur in at least
50% of PD patients who have received levodopa for 5–10 years and constitute a
major cause of disability in advanced PD. Motor fluctuations are alterations between
periods of improved mobility known as "on" periods during which the patient
responds to levodopa and periods of impaired motor function or "off" responses in
which the patient responds poorly to levodopa. As PD advances, some patients
begin experiencing wearing-off effects in which motor benefits following levodopa
are reduced in duration and last less than 4 h (the "short duration response"). The
duration of benefit after a dose of levodopa progressively shortens with disease
progression and may begin to approximate the plasma half-life of the drug, even
though levodopa plasma pharmacokinetics remain unchanged over the course of the
disease. Eventually, rare patients begin to experience rapid and unpredictable
fluctuations between "on" and "off" periods known as the "on-off" phenomenon.

Case

A 47-year-old woman with PD for 9 years was referred for consideration of deep
brain stimulation surgery. Her main problems were a progressive increase in "off"
time and the occurrence of disabling dyskinesia while she was "on." Examination
when she was "off" showed severe bilateral parkinsonism with a slow shuffling gait,
left leg tremor, and hypokinesia in all extremities. Forty-five minutes after a single
dose of levodopa, she began to display improved gait, reduced left leg tremor, and a
marked increase in finger tapping speed.

References

1. Bhidayasiri R, Truong DD. Motor complications in Parkinson's disease: clinical manifestations and management. J Neurol Sci. 2008;266:204–15.
2. Nutt JG. On-off phenomenon: relation to levodopa pharmacokinetics and pharmacodynamics.
   Ann Neurol. 1987;22:535–40.

R. Bhidayasiri, D. Tarsy, *Movement Disorders: A Video Atlas*, Current Clinical Neurology,
DOI 10.1007/978-1-60327-426-5_7, © Springer Science+Business Media New York 2012

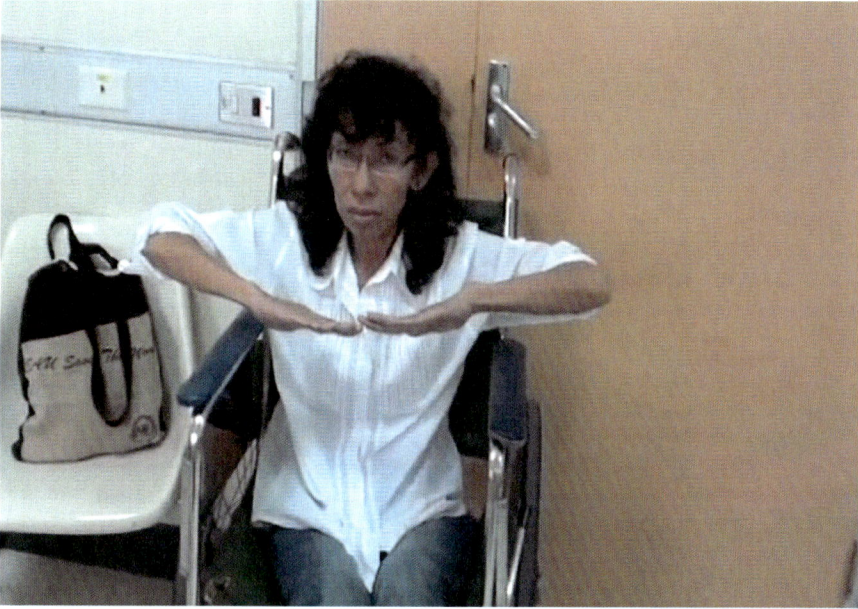

Video

During the "off" period, rapid alternating movements are relatively brisk in upper extremities and mildly slow in lower extremities. There is resting tremor in left leg. She has difficulty standing up. Gait is slow with reduced stride length and arm swing. Pull test shows retropulsion. During the "on" period, 45 min after levodopa, there is marked improvement in bradykinesia and gait, but left leg tremor persists. Heel tapping is improved. Pull test is now negative. Unified Parkinson's Disease Rating Scale motor score showed 50% improvement during the "on" period compared with the "off" period. On a different day, the patient is shown fully "on" 2 h after levodopa without leg tremor and minimal limb bradykinesia. She is able to stand up without hesitation and walks briskly with normal arm swing. She now exhibits mild truncal and extremity dyskinesia which increases while carrying out rapid upper extremity movements.

Chapter 8
Parkinson's Disease: Freezing of Gait

This chapter contains a video segment which can be found at the
URL: http://www.springerimages.com/Tarsy

Background

Freezing of gait (FOG) is also referred to as "gait ignition failure," the "slipping clutch syndrome," or "magnetic gait." FOG causes sudden but transient interruption of walking. Patients describe feeling as if their feet are "glued" or "stuck" to the floor. FOG is commonly observed while initiating gait ("start hesitation") such as after getting up from a chair or getting out of a car. It often occurs while turning when it commonly causes sudden falls. It may also be caused by a visible obstacle in the path, walking through a doorway or narrow space, in a crowded or cluttered environment, or in a situation in which the patient is rushed or startled. Once patients break free of freezing, they are very often able to walk quite normally, although FOG may also be associated with accelerating or festinating gait and/or postural instability.

FOG commonly occurs as a late manifestation of advanced Parkinson's disease (PD). It may occur during either levodopa "off" or "on" states. When present during a levodopa "on" state, it is typically unresponsive to dopaminergic therapy. FOG is also common in atypical parkinsonian syndromes including vascular parkinsonism, progressive supranuclear palsy, multiple system atrophy, and corticobasal degeneration. Two other relatively rare gait disorders are especially characterized by FOG: pure akinesia (PA) and primary progressive freezing gait (PPFG). Both syndromes are heterogeneous, but PSP appears to be the most common underlying cause of both disorders. Pharmacologic treatment is usually ineffective, except for increasing levodopa in PD when FOG occurs in the levodopa "off" state. A physiotherapy program which emphasizes sensory cueing of gait such as use of an inverted walking cane or laser cane may be helpful for patients who do not respond to routine physical and occupational therapy.

Case

A 75-year-old man with 10-year history of PD with motor fluctuations experienced increased walking difficulty. Without warning, even while in a levodopa "on" state, he would suddenly stop walking with both feet becoming stuck to the floor. An associated subjective "rushing" sensation made his symptoms worse and resulted in numerous falls. He later discovered that he was able to resume walking if he hummed a song or counted numbers out loud.

R. Bhidayasiri, D. Tarsy, *Movement Disorders: A Video Atlas*, Current Clinical Neurology,
DOI 10.1007/978-1-60327-426-5_8, © Springer Science+Business Media New York 2012

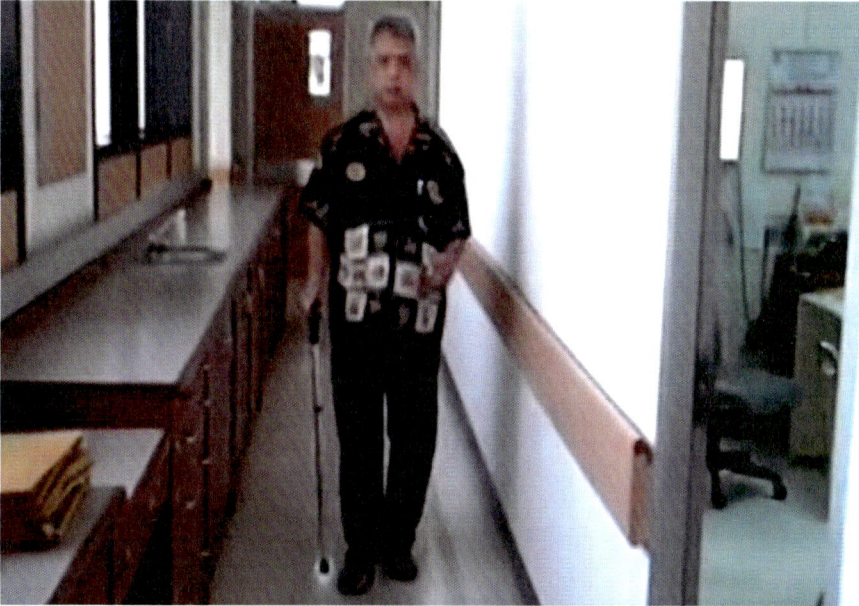

Video

Clip 1: the patient has difficulty initiating gait in a cluttered space. He exhibits start-hesitation while turning when he takes several shuffling steps. Once he breaks free of freezing, he is able to walk normally for a short distance before FOG reappears. Gait is improved while stepping over an inverted cane. Clip 2: another patient with FOG demonstrates the benefits of using a cane fitted with a crossbar across his path.

References

1. Bloem BR, Hausdorff JM, Visser JE, et al. Falls and freezing of gait in Parkinson's disease: a review of two interconnected episodic phenomena. Mov Disord. 2004;19:871–84.
2. Donovan S, Lim C, Diaz N, et al. Laser light cues for gait freezing in Parkinson's disease. Parkinsonism Relat Disord. 2011;17:240–5.
3. Fahn S. The freezing phenomenon in parkinsonism. Adv Neurol. 1995;67:53–63.

Chapter 9
Parkinsonism with Pisa Syndrome

This chapter contains a video segment which can be found at the URL: http://www.springerimages.com/Tarsy

Background

Lateral flexion of the trunk in parkinsonism, originally described as scoliosis due to parkinsonism, refers to a lateral deviation of the spine with a corresponding tendency to lean to one side which occurs in patients with relatively advanced parkinsonism. The direction of postural deviation and concavity of the scoliosis are usually contralateral to the side of greater parkinsonian signs. "Pisa syndrome" was originally used to describe a rare form of acute or tardive dystonia associated with treatment with antipsychotic drugs. The typical clinical feature is a tonic lateral flexion of the trunk associated with mild backward rotation. The head and neck may also be involved. Recently, the term "Pisa syndrome" has also been used to describe the abnormal axial posture which sometimes occurs in parkinsonism. It is a subject of debate whether lateral flexion and Pisa syndrome are the same or different conditions.

Lateral flexion of the trunk and Pisa syndrome has been reported in a number of parkinsonian disorders, particularly in idiopathic Parkinson's disease and multiple system atrophy (MSA). The sign was included as a supportive feature for the diagnosis of MSA in the second consensus statement on MSA diagnosis. The etiology of this abnormal posture is uncertain and speculatively has been attributed to several factors such as disease progression, the axial distribution of rigidity or dystonia, and possibly as effects of dopaminergic medications.

Case

A 68-year-old woman with a 10-year history of Parkinson's disease presented with increasing difficulty with ambulation. Her caregiver noticed a striking tendency to lean toward the right side which reached maximum severity over 2–3 weeks and remained unchanged during subsequent months despite adjustment of antiparkinson medications. Examination showed that the paravertebral muscles were actively contracting and hypertrophic. The patient appeared unaware of her abnormal posture.

R. Bhidayasiri, D. Tarsy, *Movement Disorders: A Video Atlas*, Current Clinical Neurology, DOI 10.1007/978-1-60327-426-5_9, © Springer Science+Business Media New York 2012

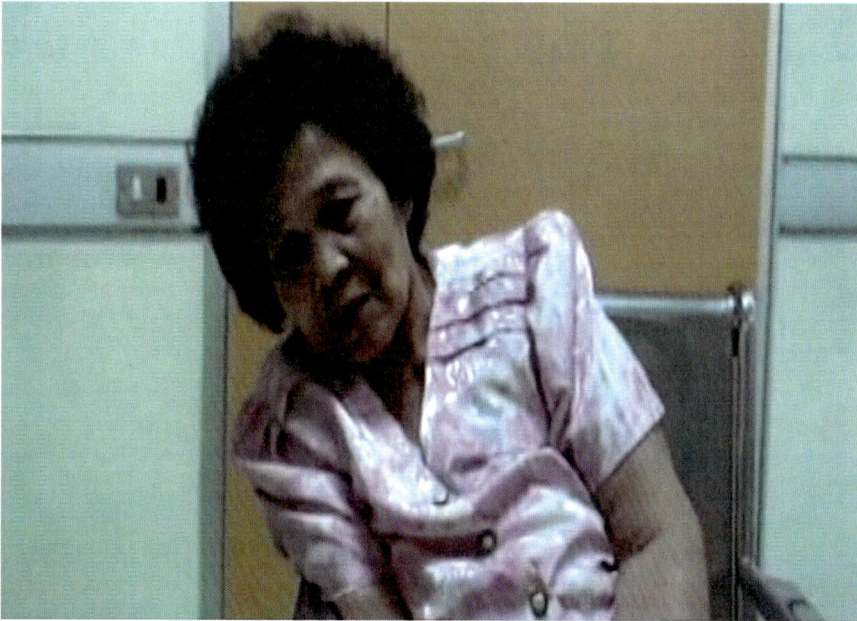

Video
Examination shows lateral flexion of the trunk to the right side while seated which is sustained and unchanged when the patient performs various motor tasks. She displays facial masking, severe hypokinesia during finger tapping, and perioral tremor.

References

1. Colosimo C. Pisa syndrome in a patient with multiple system atrophy. Mov Disord. 1998;13:607–9.
2. Di Matteo A, Fasano A, Squintani G, et al. Lateral flexion in Parkinson's disease: EMG features disclose two different underlying pathophysiological mechanism. J Neurol. 2010; 258:740–5.
3. Duvoisin RC, Marsden CD. Note on the scoliosis of parkinsonism. J Neurol Neurosurg Psychiatry. 1975;38:787–93.
4. Yokochi F. Lateral flexion in Parkinson's disease and Pisa syndrome. J Neurol. 2006;253 Suppl 7:17–20.

Chapter 10
Parkinson's Disease with Camptocormia

This chapter contains a video segment which can be found at the
URL: http://www.springerimages.com/Tarsy

Background

Camptocormia is defined as an extreme forward flexion of the thoracolumbar spine
which increases while walking and is absent in the recumbent position. The term is
an old one, originally used in World War I veterans with presumed battle stress who
developed this abnormal posture transiently without other neurological abnormalities. Currently, it is described most commonly in patients with Parkinson's disease
(PD). It can occur either early or late in the disease and usually does not correlate
with the severity of other features of parkinsonism. Patients are able to only temporarily extend their spine while standing but are immediately relieved of the symptom after reclining. It often precedes the use of levodopa and has no correlation with
levodopa-related motor fluctuations. It occurs more commonly in idiopathic PD
than multiple system atrophy and has also been reported in axial dystonia and other
basal ganglia disorders. The cause of camptocormia is uncertain. Some investiga-
tors believe it is due to dystonia of abdominal muscles, while others have presented
evidence that it is more commonly due to a myopathy of paraspinal extensor muscles. Its relationship to bent spine and dropped head syndrome in patients without
parkinsonism is unclear. Camptocormia is typically resistant to antiparkinson medications but in some cases has improved following subthalamic or globus pallidus
deep brain stimulation. Botulinum toxin injections into abdominal or iliopsoas muscles have produced only variable results.

Case

A 70-year-old man with PD presented with a 9-year history of motor symptoms
beginning with left-sided resting tremor, bradykinesia, and rigidity which evolved
over 9 years to include mild right-sided motor signs and increasingly severe camptocormia. Except for persistent camptocormia, he was initially very responsive to
levodopa with nearly complete resolution of most motor findings until end of dose
wearing off effects began 5 years after introduction of levodopa. Examination
13 years after symptom onset, while off levodopa for 12 h, showed motor UPDRS
score of 22 with mild left-sided bradykinesia and rigidity, short stride length, postural instability, and severe camptocormia unassociated with abdominal muscle dystonia or rigidity. Examination within 2 h of levodopa showed absence of tremor,
bradykinesia, and rigidity but with no change in camptocormia.

R. Bhidayasiri, D. Tarsy, *Movement Disorders: A Video Atlas*, Current Clinical Neurology,
DOI 10.1007/978-1-60327-426-5_10, © Springer Science+Business Media New York 2012

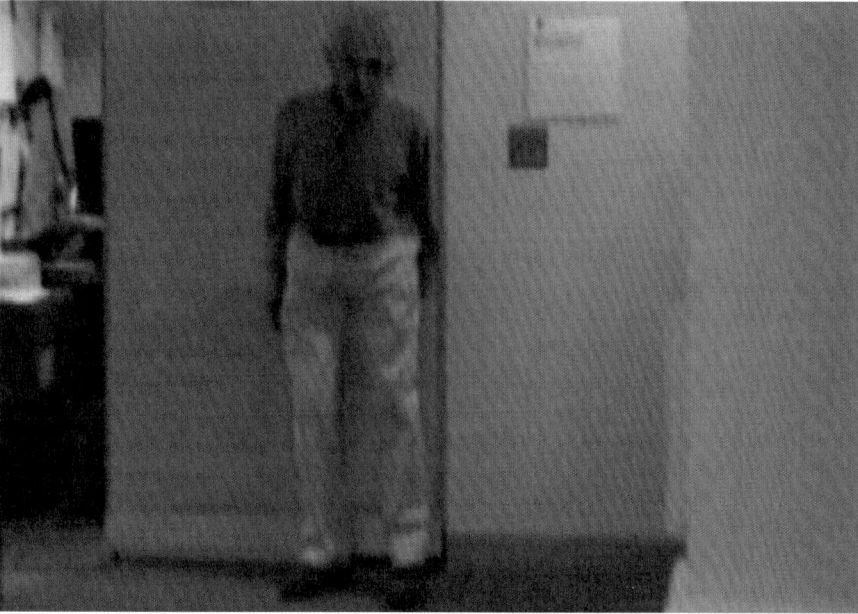

Video
Patient is in "on" state with 40° of camptocormia which is absent in a reclining position except for mildly reduced iliopsoas relaxation while reclining. Gait stability is normal except for reduced right arm swing.

References

1. Azher SN, Jankovic J. Camptocormia. Pathogenesis, classification, and response to therapy. Neurology. 2005;65:355–9.
2. Finsterer J, Strobl W. Presentation, etiology, diagnosis, and management of camptocormia. Eur Neurol. 2010;64:1–8.
3. Jankovic J. Camptocormia, head drop and other bent spine syndromes: heterogeneous etiology and pathogenesis of parkinsonian deformities. Mov Disord. 2010;25:527–8.
4. Margraf NG, Wrede A, Rohr A, et al. Camptocormia in Parkinson's disease: a focal myopathy of the paravertebral muscles. Mov Disord. 2010;25:542–51.

Chapter 11
Apathy in Parkinson's Disease

This chapter contains a video segment which can be found at the
URL: http://www.springerimages.com/Tarsy

Background

Apathy is defined as a set of behavioral, emotional, and cognitive features which are characterized by reduced interest and motivation in goal-directed behaviors, indifference, and flattened affect. While some studies focus on reduced motivation, others emphasize the lack of emotional responsiveness as a core feature. Patients typically show poor motivation with reduced initiative, effort, and perseverance as well as indifference to their circumstances. This is manifested as a lack of spontaneous engagement in or early withdrawal from their usual activities, a lack of concern for their own health, and the absence of concern for others or new experiences. A controversial issue is whether this loss of interest in goal-directed behaviors is simply the same phenomenon as the reduced interest and anhedonia characteristic of depression. In PD, apathy is commonly associated with bradyphrenia, global cognitive impairment, and executive dysfunction.

Establishing the diagnosis of apathy in PD can be challenging. Alternative explanations for loss of motivation, lack of effort, and emotional indifference may include bradykinesia, bradyphrenia, and masked facial expression. In addition, flattened affect and passivity can be manifested as hypophonia and cognitive dysfunction. Marin's criteria of reduced goal-directed behavior and the emotional concomitants of goal-directed behavior are widely used. Limited evidence suggests that dopamine deficiency, possibly involving brain limbic areas, may cause apathy and may be reversed by dopaminergic treatment. Treatment of apathy can also include nonpharmacologic strategies such as providing an individualized and structured daily schedule with varied activities. Several medications, including dopamine agonists, psychostimulants, modafinil, and testosterone, have been reported to be beneficial in small trials.

Case

A 65-year-old man with PD was seen during a follow-up visit. The family reported significant improvement in tremor and gait since initiating dopaminergic medications a year earlier. However, they noticed he was becoming increasingly passive and his initiative was becoming markedly reduced. He seemed to prefer sitting on the sofa all day with no interest in his surroundings or engaging in any activities. No tremor was present, and he was able to walk independently which was a dramatic improvement from his initial visit.

R. Bhidayasiri, D. Tarsy, *Movement Disorders: A Video Atlas*, Current Clinical Neurology,
DOI 10.1007/978-1-60327-426-5_11, © Springer Science+Business Media New York 2012

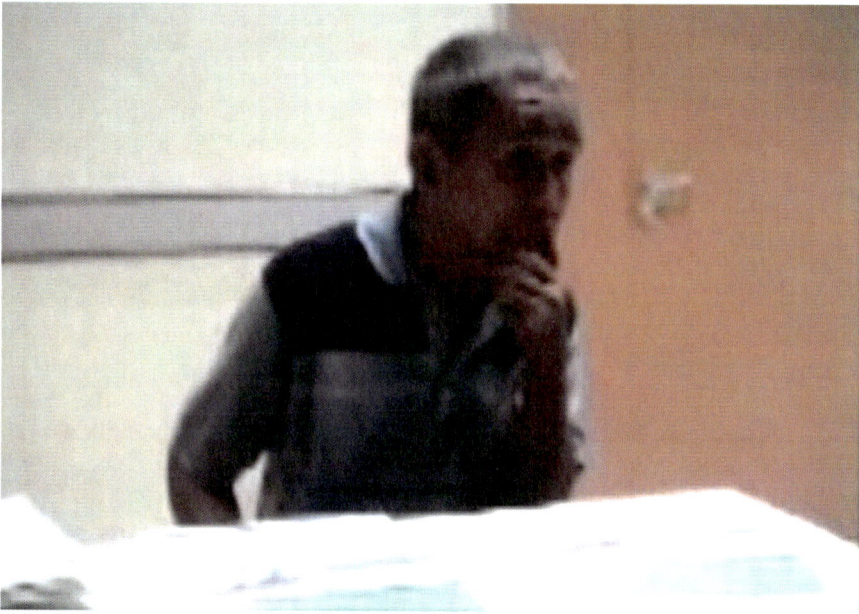

Video
The patient is very withdrawn and does not establish eye contact even when spoken to directly. He does not engage in spontaneous conversation. He sits very still with his left hand holding his chin with a significant delay before he responds to questions. When asked, he performed finger tapping and hand opening tests normally and is able to walk independently. Rigidity is minimal and no tremor is present.

References

1. Dujardin K, Sockeel P, Devos D, et al. Characteristics of apathy in Parkinson's disease. Mov Disord. 2007;22:778–84.
2. Marin RS. Differential diagnosis and classification of apathy. Am J Psychiatry. 1990;147:22–30.

Chapter 12
Punding in Parkinson's Disease

This chapter contains a video segment which can be found at the
URL: http://www.springerimages.com/Tarsy

Background

Punding, first described in amphetamine addicts, is considered to be analogous to motor
stereotypes as a continuum of behavior which ranges from excessive "hobbyism" to
prolonged, disabling, and highly stereotyped ritualistic behavior. Specific activities are
influenced by gender and individual background and include cleaning, repairing, garden-
ing, writing, artistic drawing, excessive computer or Internet use, and repeatedly catego-
rizing objects or information. Punders may neglect basic physiological needs such as
sleep, hunger, and medications. They may or may not have insight regarding the appro-
priateness of their behavior. Some patients report their activities to be soothing and may
be irritated when interrupted. Some are very agitated while carrying out their activities.

Punding has more recently been reported in patients with Parkinson's disease (PD)
being treated with dopaminergic agents, particularly dopamine agonists. The rate of
punding in the reported literature has varied between 8% and 30%. Punding appears to be
more common in patients who receive a dopaminergic medication dose of greater than
800 mg of levodopa equivalent units daily. Higher impulsivity, poorer disease-related
quality of life, younger disease onset, subthalamic nucleus deep brain stimulation (STN-
DBS), and concomitant daily medication dosage, particularly dopamine agonists, have
been found to independently predict punding-like behaviors in PD patients.

Case

A 62-year-old man who underwent subthalamic nucleus deep brain stimulation
(STN-DBS) 3 years previously was reported by his wife to be increasingly preoccupied with the task of repairing his cell phone. He would spend the entire day
working on his cell phone which his wife insisted worked perfectly well. The task
involved opening the cell phone case and taking apart the circuits and wires. He
would then put everything back together again. These tasks were carried out repeatedly several times each day, and he would become irritated if his wife reminded him
to take medications, have meals, or take a shower.

References

1. Evans AH, Katzenschlager R, Paviour D, et al. Punding in Parkinson's disease: its relation to
the dopamine dysregulation syndrome. Mov Disord. 2004;19:397–405.
2. Evans AH, Strafella AP, Weintraub D, et al. Impulsive and compulsive behaviors in Parkinson's
disease. Mov Disord. 2009;24:1561–70.

R. Bhidayasiri, D. Tarsy, *Movement Disorders: A Video Atlas*, Current Clinical Neurology,   24
DOI 10.1007/978-1-60327-426-5_12, © Springer Science+Business Media New York 2012

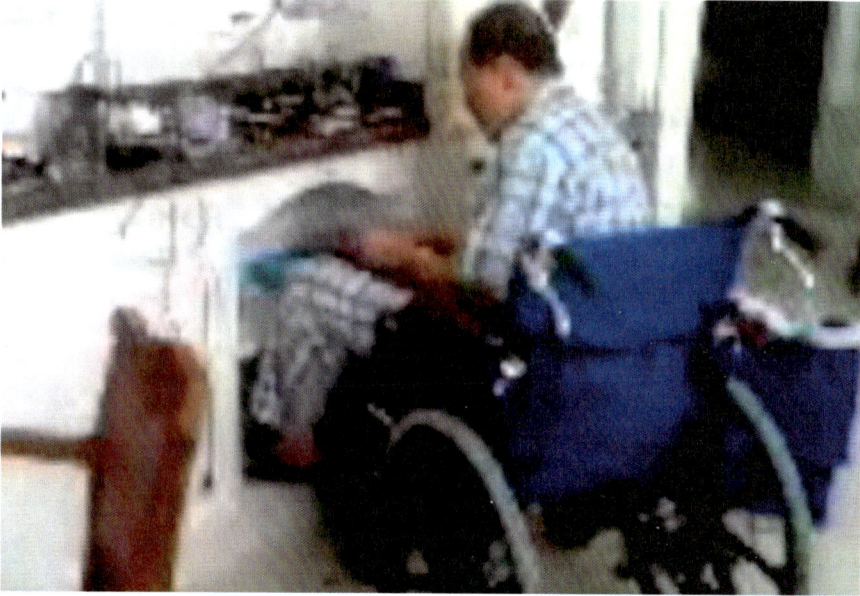

Video

The patient exhibits punding behavior manifest by being continuously preoccupied with repairing numerous cell phones. He spends more than 6 h daily manually taking apart and putting together internal parts of the cell phone.

Chapter 13
Parkinson's Disease Due to PARK2

This chapter contains a video segment which can be found at the
URL: http://www.springerimages.com/Tarsy

Background

Mutations in the parkin gene are the most frequent cause of early onset, autosomal
recessive familial Parkinson's disease (PD) and isolated juvenile-onset parkinsonism occurring before age 20. Age at onset is typically between childhood and
age 40. Patients with the parkin mutation are more likely than other PD patients to
have symmetrical involvement, focal limb dystonia, and hyperreflexia at onset.
Later they enjoy a very good response to levodopa but may develop levodopa-
induced motor fluctuations. Although the rate of progression of *PARK2*-related parkinsonism is usually relatively slow, there are no specific clinical signs which
distinguish these individuals from patients with other causes of PD. The wide spectrum of different mutations in the parkin gene renders molecular diagnosis difficult.
Pathologically, the substantia nigra undergoes severe neuronal loss and gliosis,
whereas the locus coeruleus is much less severely involved and cytoplasmic Lewy
bodies are usually absent although LB-positive cases have rarely been reported.

Case

A 67-year-old woman initially presented with a history of limping for 6 years caused
by rigidity of her left leg. There was no history of PD in her family but she was a
daughter of a consanguineous marriage. Her condition had slowly progressed for
the past 6 years. On examination, she exhibited signs of bilateral parkinsonism,
which was more severe on the left side, and a feeling of retropulsion. She responded
well to dopamine agonists and to date has not experienced motor fluctuations or
dyskinesia. There was a homozygous deletion of exons 2–4 of the parkin gene.

References

1. Kitada T, Asakawa S, Hattori N, et al. Mutations in the *parkin* gene cause autosomal recessive
   juvenile parkinsonism. Nature. 1998;392:605–8.
2. Lucking CB, Durr A, Bonifati V, et al. Association between early-onset Parkinson's disease and
   mutations in the *parkin* gene. N Eng J Med. 2000;342:1560–7.

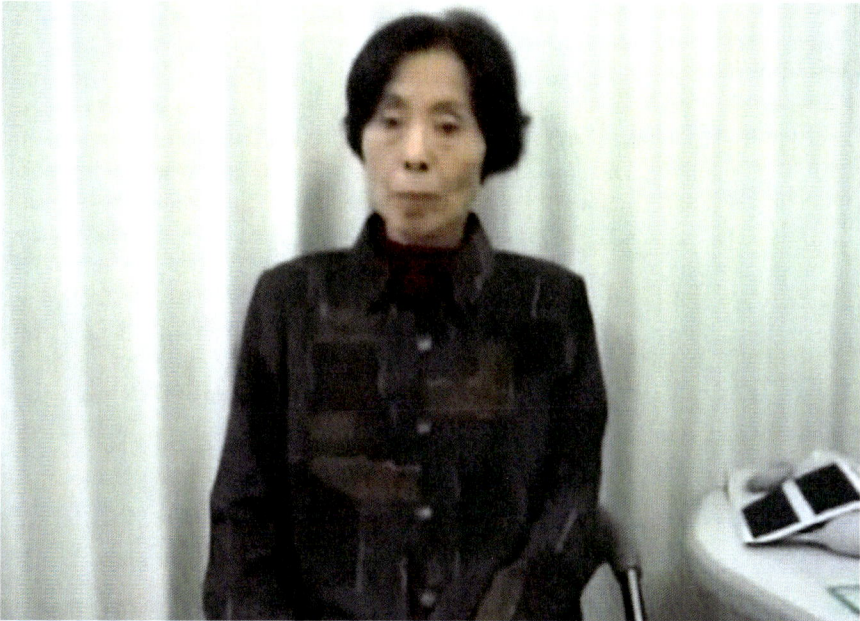

Video
Facial expression is normal. The patient displays impaired finger-tapping bilaterally. Gait is normal with reduced right arm swing. Pull testing reveals retropulsion (Video contribution from Dr. Yoshikuni Mizuno, Juntendo University School of Medicine, Tokyo, Japan).

Chapter 14
Parkinson's Disease Treated with Deep Brain Stimulation

This chapter contains a video segment which can be found at the
URL: http://www.springerimages.com/Tarsy

Background

Deep brain stimulation (DBS) is currently the surgical treatment of choice for patients with intermediate or advanced Parkinson's disease (PD) who are experiencing levodopa-related motor complications such as motor fluctuations, dyskinesias, and dystonias (see Chap. 5) which can no longer be successfully managed with antiparkinson medications. In double-blind trials, subthalamic (STN) and globus pallidus (GPi) DBS have been found to be approximately equally effective for reducing levodopa response fluctuations and improving dyskinesias in patients with advanced PD. STN-DBS allows for the dose of antiparkinson medications to be reduced, while following GPi-DBS, a direct antidyskinetic effect of DBS is achieved, but levodopa must be continued to maintain antiparkinson effects.

Case

This 32-year-old man initially presented with stiffness of his left arm and leg, incoordination of his left hand, dragging of his left leg, and difficulty turning over in bed. There was no family history of PD. Initial examination showed facial masking, markedly impaired rapid alternating movements in his left hand and foot, bilateral upper limb rigidity, and reduced armswing bilaterally. Brain MRI and tests for Wilson's disease were negative. Pramipexole was unhelpful, but he enjoyed an excellent response to the addition of levodopa/carbidopa 600 mg/day. Wearing off effects began a year after initiating levodopa and, within another year, required 100 mg doses every 3 h with entacapone for management. By 1 year later, he was reporting sudden, unpredictable wearing off with freezing episodes not consistently related to timing of doses or protein intake. A morning levodopa challenge 16 h after his last dose showed an improved UPDRS motor score from 40 to 23, followed by sudden and severe global akinesia with UPDRS motor score rising to 59. Neuropsychological testing showed mild attention deficits and executive dysfunction. Bilateral STN-DBS was carried out 4 years after his initial presentation for management of motor fluctuations. During the first 6 months of programming, his parkinsonism improved dramatically but he experienced increased levodopa dyskinesia and occasional unpredictable "off" episodes, both of which have gradually improved with multiple programming readjustments.

R. Bhidayasiri, D. Tarsy, *Movement Disorders: A Video Atlas*, Current Clinical Neurology,
DOI 10.1007/978-1-60327-426-5_14, © Springer Science+Business Media New York 2012

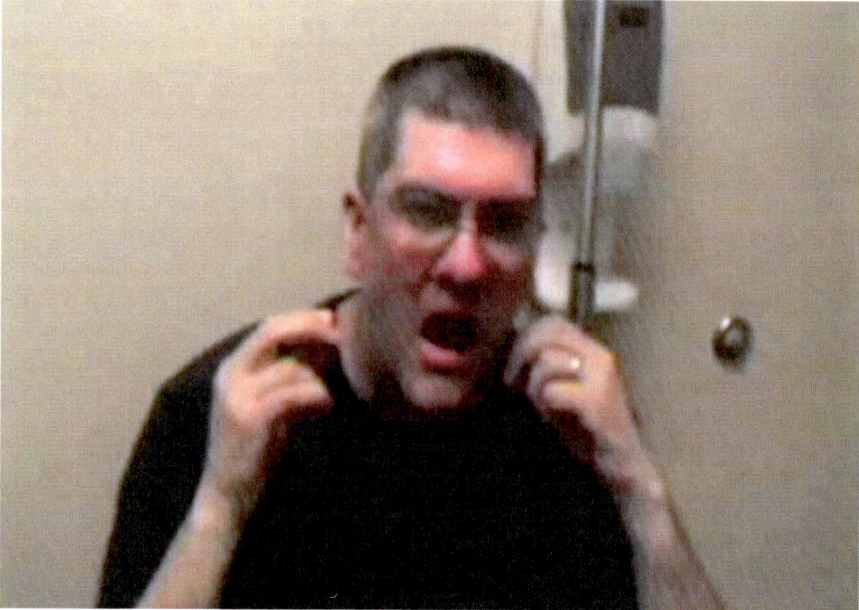

Video

Clip 1: 12 h off levodopa, with DBS off, there is severe akinesia of arms in fixed elevated position, marked facial masking, and jaw-opening dystonia. Rapid finger tapping in left hand and toe tapping in both feet are hypokinetic. Clip 2: 90 min after levodopa, with DBS on, facial masking persists but without jaw dystonia and elevation of arms. Rapid finger tapping in left hand is improved, and toe tapping is still hypokinetic. Gait is shuffling without armswing. Clip 3: on another day, while on levodopa and with DBS on, facial expression and voice are normal, gait is brisk with normal armswing, and rapid finger and hand movements are normal. (Video contribution from Dr. Ludy Shih, Beth Israel Deaconess Medical Center, Boston.)

References

1. Deuschl G, Schade-Brittinger C, Krack P, et al. A randomized trial of deep-brain stimulation for Parkinson's disease. N Engl J Med. 2006;355:896–908.
2. Weaver F, Follett K, Stern M, et al. Bilateral deep brain stimulation vs best medical therapy for patients with advanced Parkinson disease. JAMA. 2009;301:63–73.
3. Follett K, Weaver FM, Stern M, et al. Pallidal versus subthalamic deep-brain stimulation for Parkinson's disease. N Engl J Med. 2010;362:2077–91.

Chapter 15
Multiple System Atrophy

This chapter contains a video segment which can be found at the
URL: http://www.springerimages.com/Tarsy

Background

Multiple system atrophy (MSA) is an adult-onset, sporadic, progressive neurode-generative disease, characterized by varying severity of parkinsonian features, cerebellar ataxia, autonomic failure, urogenital dysfunction, and corticospinal disorders. In the past, MSA has been known as olivopontocerebellar atrophy, Shy-Drager syndrome, and striatonigral degeneration.

Consensus criteria retain the diagnostic categories of (1) MSA with predominant parkinsonism (MSA-P) and (2) MSA with predominant cerebellar ataxia (MSA-C) in order to emphasize the predominant motor features. Dysautonomia is a constant and is usually a presenting feature in both types. These criteria also retain the designations of definite, probable, and possible MSA. Definite MSA requires neuropathologic demonstration of alpha-synuclein-positive glial cytoplasmic inclusions with neurodegenerative changes in striatonigral or olivopontocerebellar structures. Probable MSA requires a sporadic, progressive, adult-onset disorder including rigorously defined autonomic failure and poorly levodopa-responsive parkinsonism or cerebellar ataxia. Possible MSA requires a sporadic, progressive adult-onset disease including parkinsonism or cerebellar ataxia, at least one feature suggesting autonomic dysfunction and one clinical or neuroimaging abnormality.

In addition to the above features, red flags supporting a clinical diagnosis of MSA include early and severe autonomic dysfunction, spontaneous or levodopa-induced orofacial dystonia, disproportionate antecollis, "Pisa syndrome," stimulus-sensitive myoclonus, dysarthria, sleep apnea, dysphagia, REM sleep behavior disorder, the "cold-hand sign," and emotional incontinence.

Case

A 55-year-old man was referred because of progressive gait instability and dysarthria. His first symptoms began 9 years earlier when his handwriting deteriorated and became smaller. He later developed stiffness in his legs and recurrent episodes of dizziness and falling. In addition, his hands became "shaky" and "jerky" as described by his colleagues at work. Initial evaluation suggested the diagnosis of idiopathic PD and he was prescribed levodopa. He reported partial improvement of his tremor but gait difficulty continued to deteriorate. Approximately 4 years previously, he broke his left wrist after a fall due to orthostatic lightheadedness.

R. Bhidayasiri, D. Tarsy, *Movement Disorders: A Video Atlas*, Current Clinical Neurology,
DOI 10.1007/978-1-60327-426-5_15, © Springer Science+Business Media New York 2012

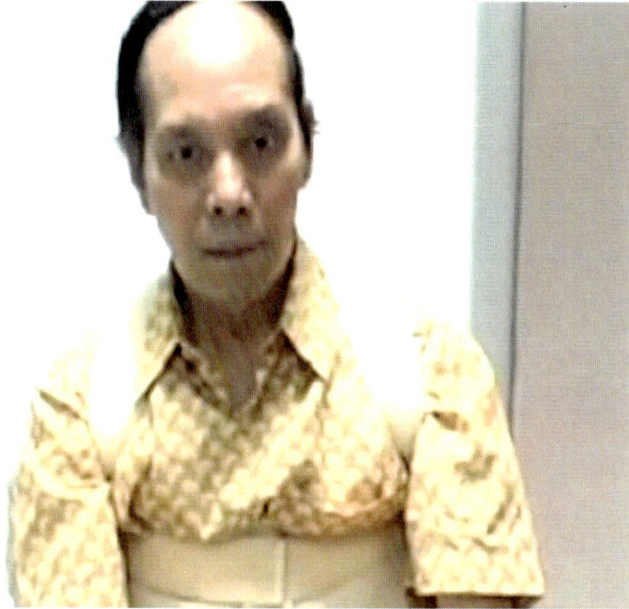

Video
The patient exhibits jerky myoclonus ("minipolymyoclonus") of the fingers with both hands outstretched. Bradykinesia is present for rapid finger tapping and hand movements. Facial masking, reduced blink frequency, global akinesia, and a mild Pisa syndrome with body tilt to the right are present.

Examination 3 h after levodopa revealed a supine blood pressure of 180/104 with pulse rate of 60/min. In upright position, systolic blood pressure dropped to 115 with a diastolic blood pressure of 39 and pulse rate of 64/min after 3 min. He became dizzy, looked pale, and needed to lie down. When he recovered, he appeared alert and communicated by pointing to letters on a card and spelling out words. Speech was limited to incomprehensible sounds. There was mild resting tremor in his right hand. Axial and extremity rigidity were present, worse on the left side. Reflexes were brisk in all extremities and extensor plantar responses were present bilaterally. He required two assistants to stand and could only walk a few small steps with a tendency to fall backward.

References

1. Bhidayasiri R, Ling H. Multiple system atrophy. Neurologist. 2008;14:224–37.
2. Gilman S, Wenning GK, Low PA, et al. Second consensus statement on the diagnosis of multiple system atrophy. Neurology. 2008;71:670–6.
3. Wenning GK, Tison F, Shlomo S, et al. Multiple system atrophy: a review of 203 pathologically proven cases. Mov Disord. 1997;12:133–47.

Chapter 16
Progressive Supranuclear Palsy

This chapter contains a video segment which can be found at the
URL: http://www.springerimages.com/Tarsy

Background

Progressive supranuclear palsy (PSP) is a clinical syndrome which includes
supranuclear gaze palsy, postural instability, and mild frontal-subcortical dementia.
PSP is characterized neuropathologically by midbrain atrophy with accumulation of
neurofibrillary tangles and glial tau pathology in a widespread topographic distribution. The most common form has been designated as Richardson's syndrome (RS)
and includes postural instability with falls, gait disorder, a supranuclear vertical
gaze palsy, eyelid opening apraxia (see Chap. 17), axial rigidity, and a frontal type
of cognitive impairment. Early clinical signs of PSP are often subtle, thereby delay-
ing the diagnosis.

In addition to classical RS, several PSP variants have been described. PSP-
parkinsonism (PSP-P) resembles Parkinson's disease (PD) and may present with
asymmetric limb rigidity, bradykinesia, and tremor with a transient response to
levodopa often leading to an erroneous diagnosis of PD. Some patients present with
a characteristic gait disturbance characterized by marked start-hesitation and gait
freezing which previously has been called "pure akinesia with gait freezing" or
"primary progressive freezing gait." Other patients with PSP have presented clinically with progressive asymmetric or unilateral dystonia, apraxia, and cortical sensory loss which has been called corticobasal syndrome (see Chap. 19). A clinical
presentation with apraxia of speech and aphasia has also been described and called
PSP-progressive nonfluent aphasia (PSP-PNFA). Common to all of these syndromes
is widespread distribution of abnormal tau protein, although the degree of tau depo-
sition appears to be greater in RS than in PSP-P.

Case

A 72-year-old man presented with recurrent falls over a period of 2 years. A diagnosis of PD was made and he was treated with levodopa on numerous occasions
without success. Examination showed slow vertical saccadic eye movements with
marked limitation of downward gaze which could be overcome with oculocephalic
maneuvers. Truncal rigidity was present without limb rigidity. His gait was lurching
with a tendency to fall backward. Pull testing was markedly positive.

R. Bhidayasiri, D. Tarsy, *Movement Disorders: A Video Atlas*, Current Clinical Neurology,
DOI 10.1007/978-1-60327-426-5_16, © Springer Science+Business Media New York 2012

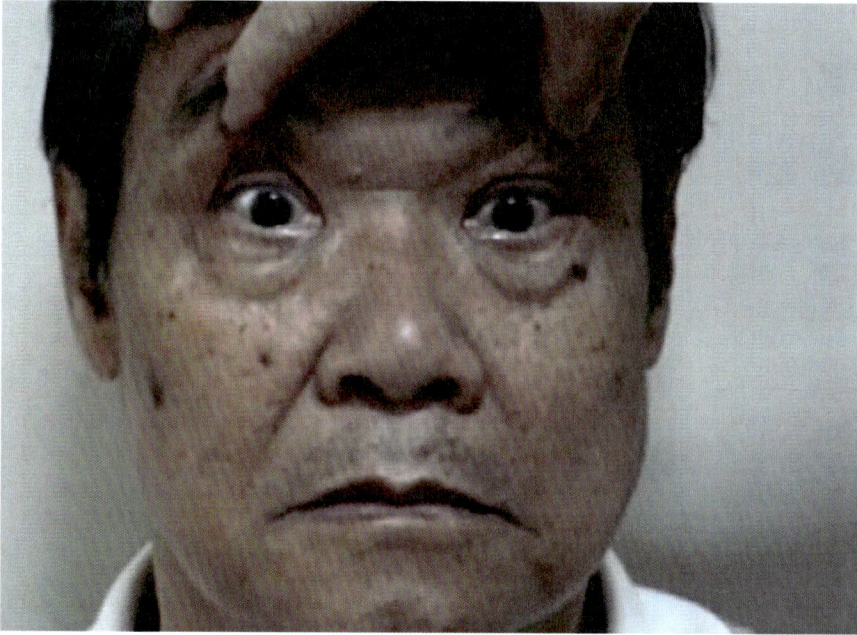

Video

Clip 1: the patient exhibits limited downward gaze and characteristic retrocollis while walking. Facial expression is absent. Gait is slow with a tendency to fall backwards when attempting to turn. Arm swing is absent bilaterally. Pull testing revealed marked postural instability. (Video contribution from Dr. Kammant Phanthumchinda, Chulalongkorn Center of Excellence on Parkinson's disease and Related Disorders, Thailand.) *Clip 2*: another patient shows nearly complete vertical and horizontal supranuclear ophthalmoplegia with relative preservation of horizontal and vertical eye movements during passive head manipulation.

References

1. Williams DR, Lees AJ. Progressive supranuclear palsy: clinicopathological concepts and diagnostic challenges. Lancet Neurol. 2009;8:270–9.
2. Williams DR, Holton JL, Strand C, et al. Pathological tau burden and distribution distinguishes progressive supranuclear palsy-parkinsonism from Richardson's syndrome. Brain. 2007;130:1566–76.
3. Bhidayasiri R, Riley DE, Somers JE, et al. Pathophysiology of slow vertical saccades in progressive supranuclear palsy. Neurology. 2001;57:2070–7.
4. Steele JC, Richardson JC, Olzewski J. Progressive supranuclear palsy. A heterogeneous degeneration involving the brain stem, basal ganglia and cerebellum with vertical supranuclear gaze and pseudobulbar palsy, nuchal dystonia and dementia. Arch Neurol. 1964;10:333–59.

Chapter 17
Progressive Supranuclear Palsy with Apraxia of Eyelid Opening

This chapter contains a video segment which can be found at the URL: http://www.springerimages.com/Tarsy

Background

Apraxia of lid opening (ALO) is a poorly recognized and highly disabling disorder which causes inability to voluntarily open the eyes. It often occurs together with blepharospasm but may also occur alone. It occurs most commonly in patients with extrapyramidal disorders, the most common of which is progressive supranuclear palsy (PSP) (see Chap. 16). It has also been associated with multiple system atrophy, Parkinson's disease, and frontal lobe injuries or stroke. Although often confused with upper eyelid ptosis, ALO occurs in the absence of lid levator weakness. The lids typically open more easily during reflex blinking and can be assisted to open by various maneuvers such as brushing the eyelids with the hand, opening the mouth, or prying open the lids with the fingers. ALO was initially attributed to involuntary levator palpebrae inhibition. However, electromyographic studies using microelectrode recordings later showed that most cases are due to persistent contraction of the pretarsal portion of the orbicularis oculi referred to as pretarsal motor persistence. Some patients appear to have a combination of levator inhibition and pretarsal motor persistence. Differential diagnosis includes essential blepharospasm in which eyelid closing is more frequent and forceful than in ALO. Ocular myasthenia gravis should also be excluded. Treatment with botulinum toxin is usually effective in cases in which pretarsal motor persistence predominates. Botulinum toxin must be injected into the pretarsal portion of orbicularis oculi immediately adjacent to the eyelashes of the upper lids in order to be effective.

Case

A 77-year-old woman presented with an 8-year history of gait disturbance, falls, and difficulty opening her eyes which was her major complaint. Examination showed slow elevation of upper eyelids with impaired ability to open her eyes, reduced speed of vertical more than horizontal saccadic eye movements, ocular square wave jerks, cervical rigidity, slow and shuffling gait, and postural instability. A diagnosis of PSP was made. Previous botulinum toxin injections into the orbital portion of orbicularis oculi had been ineffective. A series of botulinum toxin injections into pretarsal portion of orbicularis oculi as well as in lateral canthi and lower lids were given every 3 months and produced excellent relief of symptoms lasting for about 6 weeks after injections.

R. Bhidayasiri, D. Tarsy, *Movement Disorders: A Video Atlas*, Current Clinical Neurology, DOI 10.1007/978-1-60327-426-5_17, © Springer Science+Business Media New York 2012

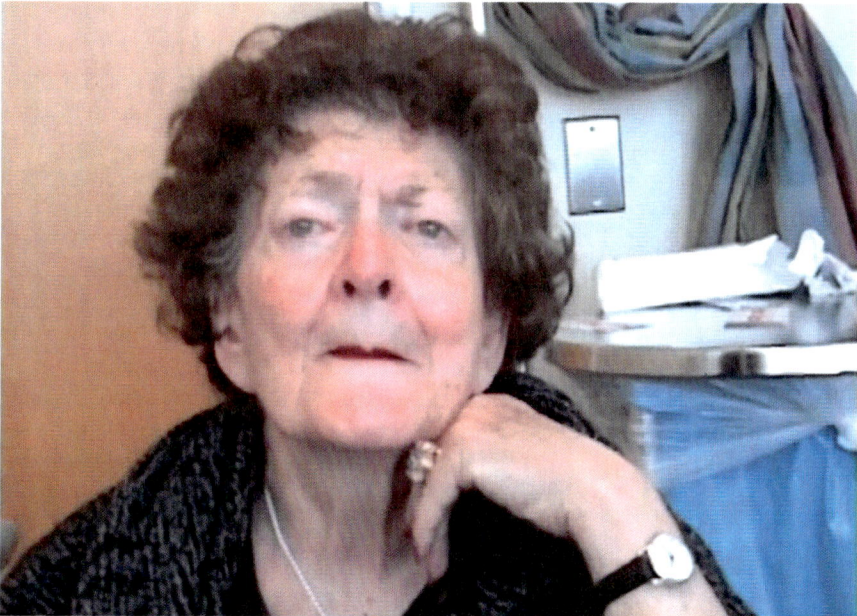

Video
The patient exhibits slow voluntary elevation of upper eyelids, slow saccadic eye movements involving vertical more than horizontal gaze and, at the time of this video, only mild hesitation opening her eye due to recent treatment with botulinum toxin. Other features of PSP include hyperextension of the neck, facial masking, and monotonic voice.

References

1. Elston JS. A new variant of blepharospasm. J Neurol Neurosurg Psychiatry. 1992;55:369–71.
2. Aramideh M, de Ongerboer Visser BW, Koelman JHTM, et al. Clinical and electromyographic features of levator palpebrae superioris muscle dysfunction in involuntary eyelid closure. Mov Disord. 1994;9:395–402.
3. Boghen D. Apraxia of lid opening: a review. Neurology. 1997;48:1491–503.

Chapter 18
Vascular Parkinsonism

This chapter contains a video segment which can be found at the
URL: http://www.springerimages.com/Tarsy

Background

Vascular parkinsonism (VP), originally known as arteriosclerotic parkinsonism, is a
heterogeneous but clinically recognizable entity which is comprised of predominantly "lower body parkinsonism," postural instability, and falls. In comparison
with Parkinson's disease (PD), patients with VP tend to be older, have a shorter
duration of illness, may have a stepwise decline, present with symmetrical gait
difficulties, are less responsive to levodopa, and are more prone to postural instability, falls, and dementia. Pyramidal signs, pseudobulbar palsy, and incontinence are
commonly present. While no specific abnormal structural imaging pattern is suggestive of VP, brain CT and MRI often demonstrate evidence of vascular impairment with frequent involvement of more than one vascular territory and abnormalities
in periventricular and subcortical white matter and basal ganglia. The clinical criteria for diagnosis of VP have been proposed as follows: bradykinesia involving
mainly the lower extremities associated with reduced stride length and at least one
of the following: resting tremor, rigidity, and postural instability; the presence of
cerebrovascular disease supported by brain CT or MRI and/or clinical examination
confirming focal signs or symptoms compatible with a stroke or strokes, and a relationship between the above disorders including an acute presentation of parkinsonism with multiple infarcts in or near basal ganglia or a more insidious onset with
extensive subcortical white matter lesions.

Case

A 75-year-old man with a history of hypertension and diabetes mellitus presented
with a 2-year history of progressive gait difficulty. His steps had become smaller
and he tended to fall when attempting to turn. Sometimes he felt as if his feet were
glued to the floor, making it impossible for him to start walking. Examination
revealed only mild signs of parkinsonism in the upper extremities but foot tapping
was impaired, stride length was short, and gait was characterized by hesitation,
shuffling, and occasional unpredictable freezing of gait. Reflexes were hyperactive
in the lower extremities with bilateral extensor plantar responses. Brain MRI
showed a moderate degree of small vessel disease in the periventricular white matter and small lacunar infarcts in the right basal ganglia without evidence of
hydrocephalus.

R. Bhidayasiri, D. Tarsy, *Movement Disorders: A Video Atlas*, Current Clinical Neurology,
DOI 10.1007/978-1-60327-426-5_18, © Springer Science+Business Media New York 2012

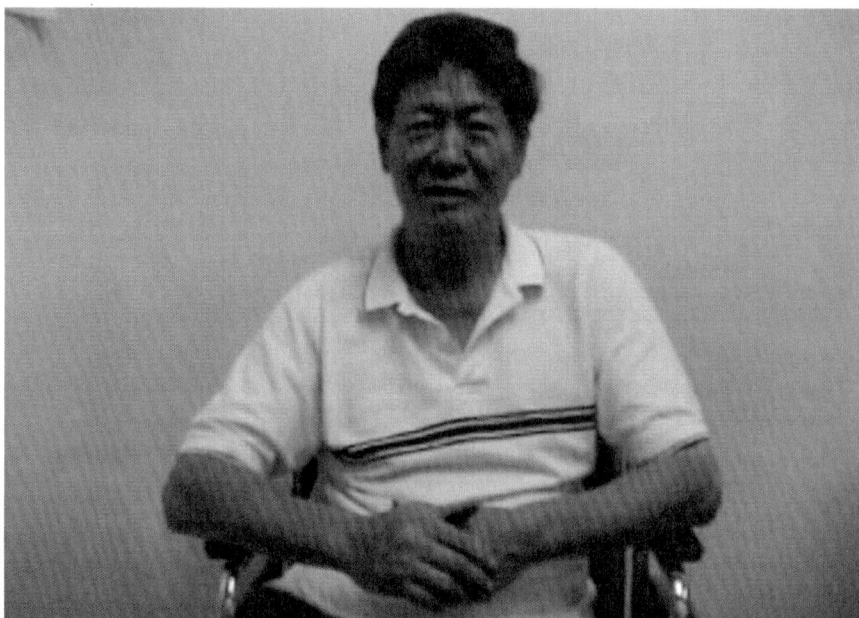

Video

Motor examination reveals relatively mild parkinsonism in upper extremities. Voice is hypophonic and monotonic. Signs of parkinsonism predominantly affect the lower extremities with short stride length, shuffling gait, and occasional freezing of gait. Freezing of gait could be overcome by stepping over obstacles. Pull testing is positive.

References

1. Winnikates J, Jankovic J. Clinical correlates of vascular parkinsonism. Arch Neurol. 1999; 56:98–102.
2. Zijlmans JCM, Daniel SE, Hughes AJ, et al. Clinicopathological investigation of vascular parkinsonism, including clinical criteria for diagnosis. Mov Disord. 2004;19:630–40.

Chapter 19
Corticobasal Degeneration

This chapter contains a video segment which can be found at the
URL: http://www.springerimages.com/Tarsy

Background

Corticobasal degeneration (CBD) is a clinically heterogeneous disorder associated
with characteristic neuropathologic findings. These include cortical and nigral atrophy, numerous swollen cortical neurons, and tau-immunoreactive astrocytic plaques
which are not present in other tauopathies. Classically, CBD patients present in the
sixth to eighth decade with a myriad of motor manifestations including limb dystonia, focal reflex myoclonus, postural/action tremor, and akinetic rigidity; cerebral
cortical deficits including cortical sensory loss, apraxia, an alien limb phenomenon,
and aphasia; and other clinical features such as oculomotor apraxia and corticospinal tract signs.

Contrary to earlier descriptions, asymmetry of clinical findings is common but is
not always present, particularly in individuals presenting with frontal cognitive
deficits. There is so much variability between the clinical presentation and final
neuropathological findings that the concept of a corticobasal syndrome (CBS) has
emerged in which patients with a constellation of clinical findings suggestive of
CBD may turn out to have neuropathological evidence for other disorders such as
frontotemporal dementia, progressive supranuclear palsy (PSP), and Alzheimer's
disease. In addition, patients with evidence for CBD at postmortem may in life have
exhibited a heterogeneous clinical picture including frontotemporal dementia, progressive non-fluent aphasia, a PSP-like syndrome, and a posterior cortical atrophy
syndrome.

Case

A 75-year-old woman presented with progressive stiffness and a 2-year history of
right arm jerking. Initially, her right arm had become clumsy and was severely painful whenever it was touched. Symptoms gradually progressed to include slowness
of body movements and frequent falls. Examination showed a fixed flexion dystonia
of her right arm and hand associated with marked rigidity. Global hypokinesia was
present which was more pronounced on the right side. Due to the severe right arm
dystonia, it was impossible to assess for apraxia. Allodynia was present in the right
arm. She was unable to walk due to stiffness of both legs.

R. Bhidayasiri, D. Tarsy, *Movement Disorders: A Video Atlas*, Current Clinical Neurology,
DOI 10.1007/978-1-60327-426-5_19, © Springer Science+Business Media New York 2012

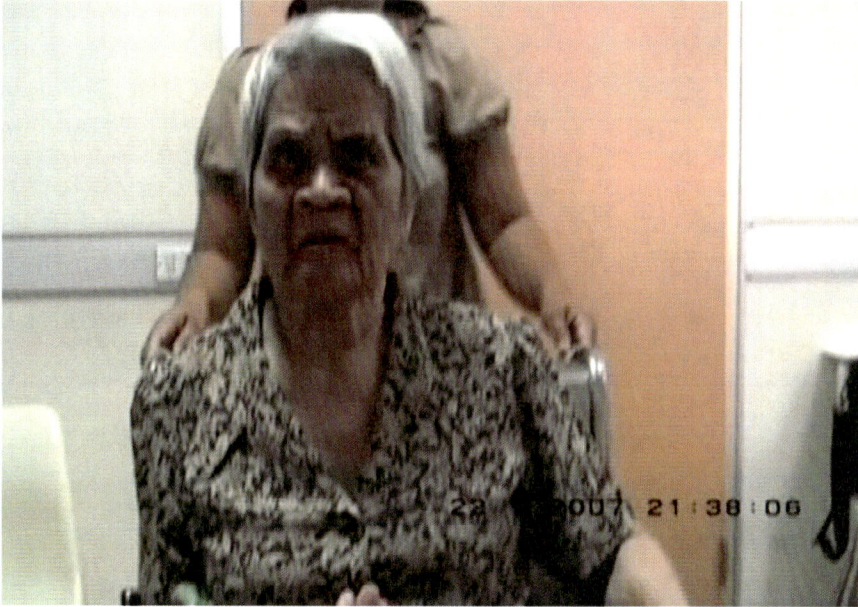

Video *Clip 1*: this patient with CBS exhibits dystonia with a fixed adducted and flexed posture of her right arm, hand, and fingers. When testing for apraxia, the patient was able to show her left arm and left two fingers. She was unable to perform these tasks on the right side due to the severe dystonia. She was able to locate her right arm with her left hand. *Clip 2*: another patient with CBS displays a fixed, dystonic posture of the right hand.

References

1. Boeve BF, Lang AE, Litvan I. Corticobasal degeneration and its relationship to progressive supranuclear palsy and frontotemporal dementia. Ann Neurol. 2003;53 Suppl 5:S15–9.
2. Ludolph AC, Kassubek J, Landwehrmeyer BG, et al. Tauopathies with parkinsonism: clinical spectrum, neuropathologic basis, biological markers, and treatment options. Eur J Neurol. 2009;16:297–309.
3. Ling H, O'Sullivan SS, Holton JL, et al. Does corticobasal degeneration exist? A clinicopathological re-evaluation. Brain. 2010;133:2045–57.
4. Lee SE, Rabinovici GD, Mayo MC, et al. Clinicopathological correlations in corticobasal degeneration. Ann Neurol. 2011;70:327–40.

Chapter 20
Drug-Induced Parkinsonism

This chapter contains a video segment which can be found at the
URL: http://www.springerimages.com/Tarsy

Background

Drug-induced parkinsonism (DIP) is a common adverse effect of treatment with
antipsychotic/neuroleptic drugs which block dopamine receptors in the striatum.
These drugs include the phenothiazines, thioxanthenes, butyrophenones, and the
newer-generation "atypical" antipsychotic drugs such as risperidone, olanzapine,
ziprasidone, and aripiprazole. Antiemetics which block dopamine receptors such as
prochlorperazine and metoclopramide and certain calcium channel blockers such as
flunarizine are also common causes of DIP. DIP may be indistinguishable from
Parkinson's disease (PD) and includes various combinations of bradykinesia, rigidity, resting and action tremor. The incidence of DIP increases with age. In fact,
asymmetric motor findings are not uncommon and in older individuals may represent an unmasking of subclinical PD. No diagnostic tests are available, although
PET studies will show normal striatal F-dopa uptake unless subclinical PD is present. Treatment consists of either lowering the dose or changing to those atypical
antipsychotic drugs which do not cause DIP such as clozapine or quetiapine.
Treatment with amantadine may be helpful, but anticholinergic drugs and levodopa
are ineffective and may exacerbate psychiatric symptoms.

Case

This 69-year-old left-handed man with hypertension and coronary artery disease presented with left-sided hemichorea and hemiballismus which evolved over 7 days (see
Chap. 75). Examination showed intermittent left-sided choreiform and ballistic movements. Brain CT and MRI both showed hyperintensity of the right putamen and caudate which cleared gradually over 1 month without signs of infarction or hemorrhage.
He was placed on haloperidol 12 mg daily and within 10 days developed obvious signs
of parkinsonism with facial masking, hypophonia, generalized bradykinesia, and mild
focal bradykinesia and rigidity in right upper extremity. Gait was slow with reduced
stride length and absent right arm swing. Mild residual left hemichorea remained evident. Haloperidol was stopped and signs of parkinsonism cleared over 10 days with
increased left hemichorea/hemiballismus. He was placed on tetrabenazine with
improvement in hemichorea but the reappearance of mild parkinsonism together with
depression. Tetrabenazine was stopped and later reintroduced at a lower dose together
with citalopram with satisfactory control of hemichorea and depression.

R. Bhidayasiri, D. Tarsy, *Movement Disorders: A Video Atlas*, Current Clinical Neurology,
DOI 10.1007/978-1-60327-426-5_20, © Springer Science+Business Media New York 2012

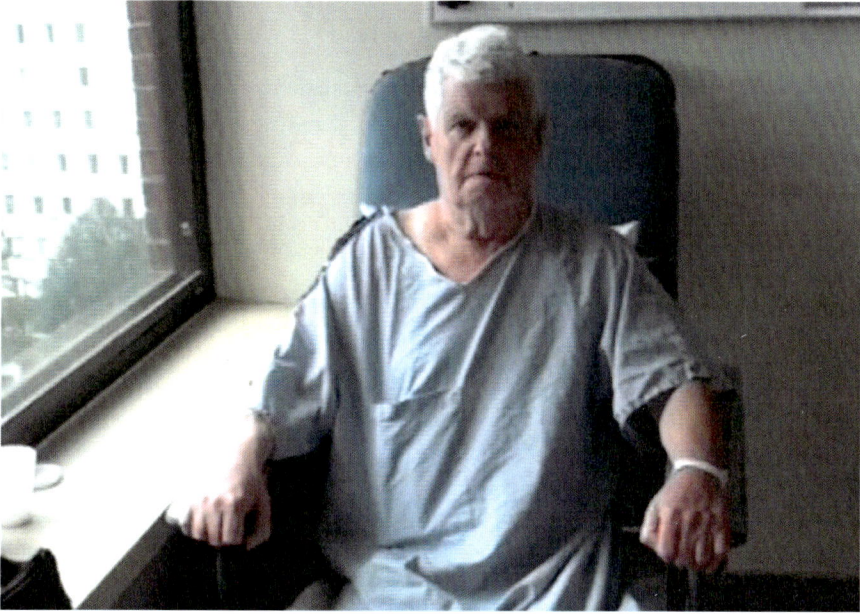

Video
Patient is in hospital displaying facial masking, reduced blink frequency, global bradykinesia, slow and hypokinetic right finger and toe tapping, and slow gait with flexed posture, absent arm swing and en bloc turns following 10 days of treatment with haloperidol for hemiballismus (see Chap. 75).

References

1. Tarsy D. Movement disorders with neuroleptic drug treatment. Psych Clin North Am. 1984; 7:453–71.
2. Chabolla DR, Maraganore DM, Ahlskog JE, et al. Drug-induced parkinsonism as a risk factor for Parkinson's disease: a historical cohort study in Olmsted county, Minnesota. Mayo Clin Proc. 1998;73:724–7.
3. Burn DJ, Brooks DJ. Nigral dysfunction in drug-induced parkinsonism: an ^{18}F-dopa PET study. Neurology. 1993;43:552–6.

Chapter 21
Toxin-Induced Parkinsonism

This chapter contains a video segment which can be found at the
URL: http://www.springerimages.com/Tarsy

Background

Parkinsonism has been reported to occur due to a number of toxins including metals
(iron, copper, and manganese), the by-product 1-methyl-4-phenyl-1,2,3,6-tetrahy-
dropyridine (MPTP), and certain pesticides, such as paraquat, organochlorine, and
carbamate. The specific mechanisms by which these neurotoxins damage nigral
dopaminergic neurons are unknown. An important mechanism by which neurotoxins could selectively target dopaminergic cells may be via uptake through the presynaptic dopamine transporter. Because of the potential role of pesticides as an
environmental risk factor for Parkinson's disease (PD), several paradigms have been
developed to create animal models of PD including MPTP, 6-hydroxydopamine,
and rotenone. Despite clinical similarities, the principal differences between PD and
these animal models are the lack of progressive neurodegeneration and the absence
of typical neuronal Lewy bodies in the animal models. In humans, clinical and pathological studies involving patients with parkinsonism following exposure to these
toxins are lacking. Clinical presentations appear to be heterogeneous but most commonly have included akinetic-rigid parkinsonism, prominent postural instability,
and dystonia.

Case

A 35-year-old man was admitted to an intensive care unit following ingestion of a
large quantity of pesticides of unknown type. While regaining consciousness, he
exhibited marked bilateral symmetric parkinsonism with facial masking, blepharospasm, and rigidity and hypokinesia of all four extremities without tremor. Brain
MRI was normal. He responded partially to levodopa with decreased rigidity and
akinesia. Blepharospasm responded to botulinum toxin injections. However, he
was left with significant permanent disability due to impaired limb dexterity and
significant rigidity.

R. Bhidayasiri, D. Tarsy, *Movement Disorders: A Video Atlas*, Current Clinical Neurology,
DOI 10.1007/978-1-60327-426-5_21, © Springer Science+Business Media New York 2012

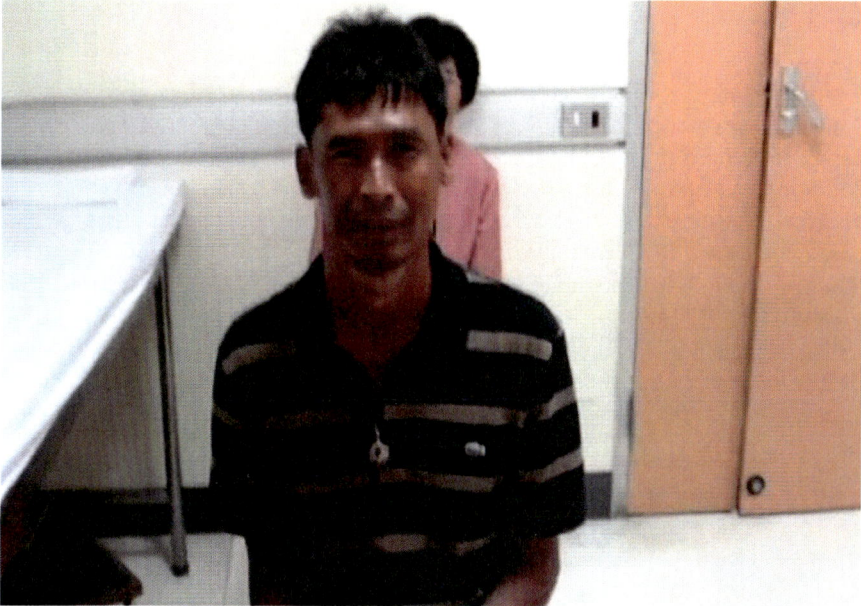

Video
The patient exhibits signs of akinetic-rigid parkinsonism with severe facial masking and increased blink frequency. He displays bilateral hand dystonia and marked left-sided hypokinesia. His gait is associated with absent left arm swing.

References

1. Di Monte DA. The environmental and Parkinson's disease: Is the nigrostriatal system preferentially targeted by neurotoxins? Lancet Neurol. 2003;2:531–8.
2. Langston JW, Ballard P, Tetrud JW, et al. Chronic parkinsonism in humans due to a product of meperidine-analog synthesis. Science. 1983;219:979–80.
3. Bhatt MM, Elias MA, Mankodi MA, et al. Acute and reversible parkinsonism due to organophosphate pesticide intoxication: five cases. Neurology. 1999;52:1467–71.

Chapter 22
HIV-Induced Parkinsonism

This chapter contains a video segment which can be found at the URL: http://www.springerimages.com/Tarsy

Background

Parkinsonism is the most common movement disorder to affect HIV-infected patients and occurs in 5% of cases. Parkinsonism often occurs in the context of prior exposure to neuroleptic drugs, focal cerebral opportunistic infections, or HIV/AIDS-associated dementia. AIDS patients have a 2.4–3.4-fold greater risk of developing extrapyramidal side effects when they are exposed to neuroleptic drugs. The basal ganglia are a vulnerable target to HIV, and parkinsonism may develop in the absence of any other identifiable underlying cause. The clinical features of HIV parkinsonism are usually different than those of idiopathic Parkinson's disease (PD) in that they include bilateral onset, rapid progression, abnormal eye movements, and no rest tremor. However, in some patients, HIV parkinsonism may be clinically similar to idiopathic PD but differentiated by rapid symptom progression and earlier development of motor complications. Most patients report clinical improvement with highly active antiretroviral therapy.

Case

A 45-year-old female who had been HIV seropositive for several years was referred due to a bizarre gait and slow movements. The patient had stopped her antiretroviral regimen a few months previously, apparently due to lack of follow-up. Examination showed facial masking, mild drooling, and bradykinesia with rigidity in both upper extremities. No tremor was present. Her gait was wide-based and she walked on her toes. She was slow to respond to verbal commands. Brain MRI showed mild generalized cerebral atrophy without focal lesions.

References

1. Mirsattari SM, Power C, Nath A. Parkinsonism with HIV infection. Mov Disord. 1998; 13:684–9.
2. Tse W, Cersosimo MG, Gracies JM, et al. Movement disorders and AIDS: a review. Parkinsonism Relat Disord. 2004;10:323–34.

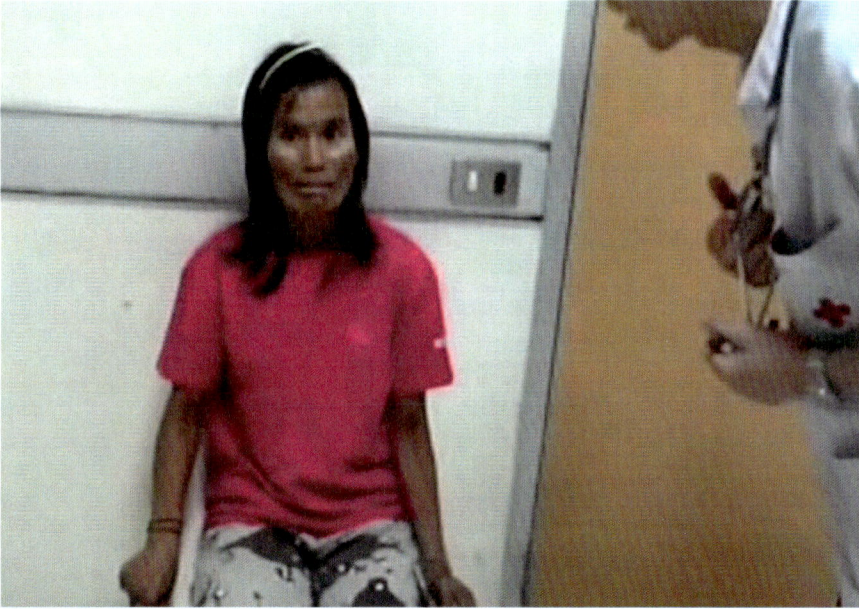

Video
The patient displays generalized bradykinesia and facial masking with reduced blink frequency. Tongue movements are slow. Finger tapping is slow with reduced amplitude bilaterally. Gait is wide-based and arm swing is present.

Part II
Tremor

Chapter 23
Examination of a Patient with Essential Tremor

This chapter contains a video segment which can be found at the
URL: http://www.springerimages.com/Tarsy

Background

Essential tremor (ET) is the most common cause of postural and kinetic tremor arising
from a primary neurologic disorder with an estimated worldwide prevalence of 5%.
The incidence of ET increases with age but often affects young individuals. ET is also
referred to as familial tremor when there is a family history which is present in about
50% of cases. ET appears to be genetically heterogeneous. Although genetic linkage
studies have discovered a genetic basis for ET in several affected families, the genetic
basis for ET has not been identified in the vast majority of cases. The pathological
basis for ET remains uncertain, although postmortem cerebellar Purkinje cell abnormalities have been found in some patients. ET most often affects the upper extremities
but may also affect the head, voice, trunk, and legs. ET is a highly heterogeneous
disorder with variations in tremor frequency, topographic distribution, and severity.
Most commonly, ET causes a postural tremor of the extended arms and hands but
often appears as a large amplitude kinetic tremor which increases during or at the very
end of goal-directed movements such as drinking from a glass or eating from a spoon.
By definition, tremor is the only manifestation of ET, although in severe cases there
may be an associated gait disorder. Differential diagnosis of tremor includes parkinsonian tremor which, in some cases, can be associated with significant postural tremor
(see Chap. 24), tremor associated with other neurological disorders, primary writing
tremor (see Chap. 29), and enhanced physiologic tremor (see Chap. 31). Propranolol
or other beta-blockers and primidone are the most effective pharmacologic treatments
for ET. Other anticonvulsants which are sometimes effective in ET include topiramate, gabapentin, and zonisamide. Although small amounts of alcohol produce temporary relief of ET in some patients, its effect is relatively brief and may be associated
with a rebound increase in tremor afterward. Thalamic deep brain stimulation is very
effective for medically refractory ET.

Case

A 54-year-old man first developed hand tremor in childhood. This gradually progressed throughout adulthood and intensified during the past 2 years. It has disturbed
writing, eating, drinking, and using a computer mouse. Tremor was markedly relieved
by small amounts of alcohol. Caffeine and bronchodilators did not aggravate the
tremor. There was no voice or head tremor. There was no family history of tremor.

R. Bhidayasiri, D. Tarsy, *Movement Disorders: A Video Atlas*, Current Clinical Neurology,   48
DOI 10.1007/978-1-60327-426-5_23, © Springer Science+Business Media New York 2012

Examination showed relatively mild postural tremor of his extended hands with more severe right hand tremor in the "wing-beating" posture and while drawing, drinking from a paper cup, and pouring water. Examination was otherwise normal. Topiramate and gabapentin were unhelpful and he declined beta-blockers because of asthma. Primidone 250 mg daily was helpful in partially reducing tremor severity.

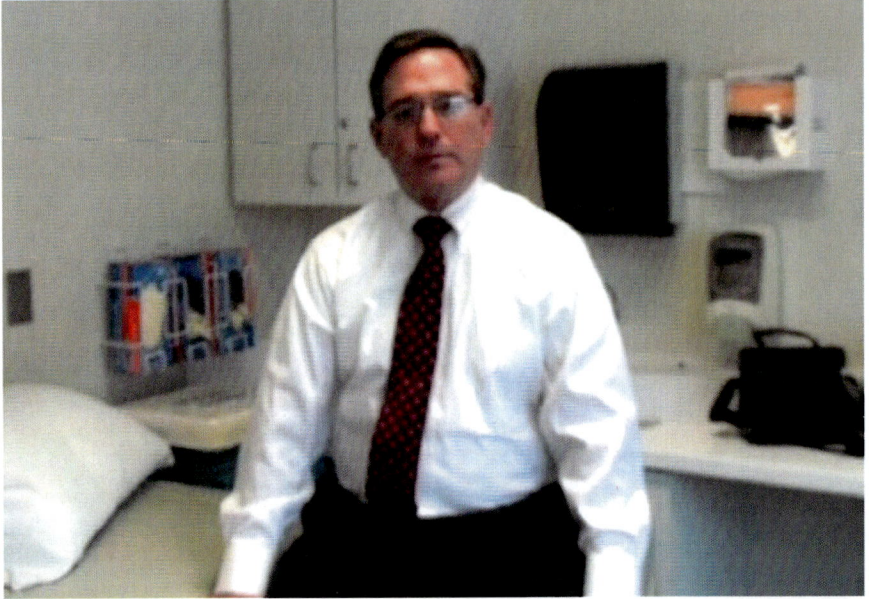

Video

Clip 1: the patient is examined using the essential tremor rating assessment scale (TETRAS). He displays mild postural tremor of his extended hands, delayed appearance of large amplitude tremor of right hand in the "wing-beating" posture, a tremor drawing spirals with his left hand more affected than the right hand, tremor positioning a pen point above a target, and writing tremor. *Clip 2*: another patient with ET is examined using TETRAS. He exhibits voice tremor, head tremor, and tremor of his hands while extended and in the wing-beating position. Drawing of a spiral, positioning a pen point above a target, and writing are all tremulous.

References

1. Louis ED. Clinical practice. Essential tremor. N Engl J Med. 2001;345:887–91.
2. Jankovic J. Essential tremor: a heterogeneous disorder. Mov Disord. 2002;17:638–44.
3. Ondo W, Jankovic J. Essential tremor: treatment options. CNS Drugs. 1996;6:178–91.
4. Elble R, Comella C, Fahn S, the Tremor Research Group. The essential tremor rating assessment scale (TETRAS). Mov Disord. 2008;23 Suppl 1:S357.

Chapter 24
Parkinsonian Rest, Postural, and Re-emergent Tremor

This chapter contains a video segment which can be found at the
URL: http://www.springerimages.com/Tarsy

Background

Rest tremor is generally regarded as the characteristic tremor which is associated
with Parkinson's disease (PD). However, some patients with PD also experience a
postural tremor which may be unilateral or bilateral and may be more severe and
disabling than their rest tremor. If other signs of PD are not yet present, a misdiag-
nosis of essential tremor (ET) is often made. The postural tremor of ET occurs
immediately after the upper limbs are raised to a horizontal position, while the postural tremor of PD occurs after a latency of about 5 s and has the same frequency as
the patient's rest tremor. The latter is referred to as re-emergent tremor. The amplitude of postural tremor in PD is usually larger than in ET. Unlike ET, the re-emergent
tremor of PD may respond to antiparkinson medications. Re-emergent tremor is
more disabling than rest tremor and in severe cases has been successfully treated
with thalamic deep brain stimulation (DBS).

Case

A 64-year-old man presented with a 4-year history of right lower extremity rest
tremor and a fine postural tremor of both hands followed 2 years later by right upper
extremity rest tremor. More recently, right upper extremity tremor began occurring
while using his right hand and arm and as a result became increasingly disabling.
A diagnosis of ET had been made several years previously but treatments with propranolol and primidone were unhelpful. Examination showed intermittent rest
tremor in right hand and continuous rest tremor in right leg. Tremor in the right arm
disappeared when extended horizontally before it reappeared within several seconds and became much larger in amplitude. Tremor was absent during quick finger-
nose-finger movements, while drinking from a cup, and pouring. The rest and
postural tremors both increased with mental distraction maneuvers. Right arm swing
was reduced, and there was slight focal bradykinesia and rigidity in right hand.
Handwriting was micrographic. Trials of trihexyphenidyl, zonisamide, and levodopa
were unhelpful. Left subthalamic DBS was carried out 6 months after presentation
and successfully alleviated all manifestations of tremor in right arm and leg.

R. Bhidayasiri, D. Tarsy, *Movement Disorders: A Video Atlas*, Current Clinical Neurology,
DOI 10.1007/978-1-60327-426-5_24, © Springer Science+Business Media New York 2012

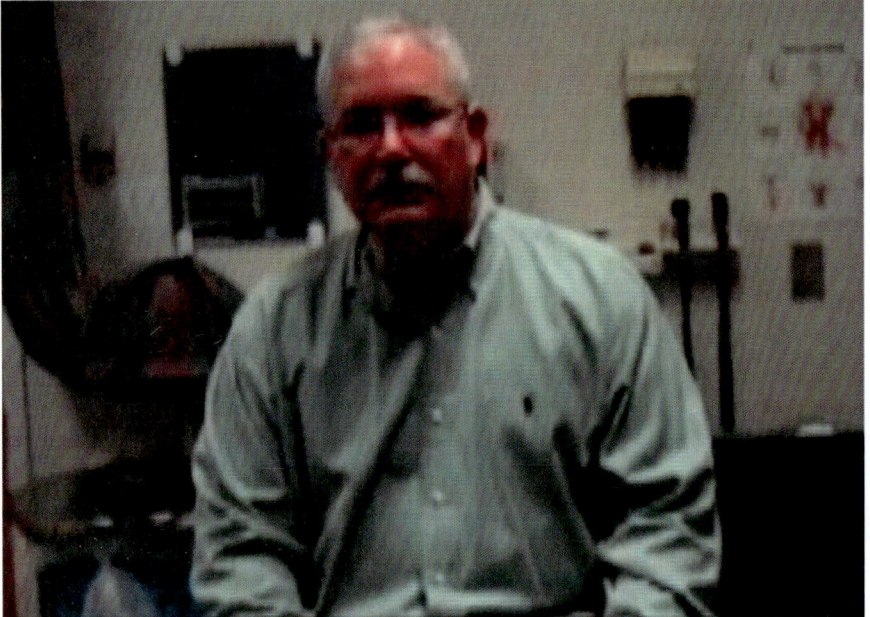

Video

The patient shows continuous rest tremor in left arm and leg. With arms extended, the right arm tremor improves and then reappears while he recites the months of the year. It later appears spontaneously just prior to being asked to recite months of year backward a second time.

References

1. Jankovic J, Schwartz KS, Ondo W. Re-emergent tremor of Parkinson's disease. J Neurol Neurosurg Psychiatry. 1989;67:646–50.
2. Tarsy D, Scollins L, Corapi K, O'Herron S, Apetauerova D, Norregaard T. Progression of Parkinson's disease following thalamic deep brain stimulation for tremor. Stereotact Funct Neurosurg. 2006;83:222–7.

Chapter 25
Essential Tremor: Voice and Head Tremor

This chapter contains a video segment which can be found at the
URL: http://www.springerimages.com/Tarsy

Background

Essential tremor (ET) is a monosymptomatic disorder that is most commonly characterized by a postural and kinetic tremor of the upper extremities which is often
accompanied by head and voice tremor (see Chap. 23). In some patients, voice and
head tremor predominate and can be the most apparent and disturbing manifestations of ET. The head tremor may be vertical ("yes-yes"), horizontal ("no-no"),
rotatory, or mixed. Head tremor is rhythmic and typically continuous, showing very
little change with alterations in head position. In milder cases, patients are often
unaware of head tremor. Voice tremor produces tremulous and wavering speech
without major dysarthria. Differential diagnosis of head tremor includes the dystonic head tremor of cervical dystonia (spasmodic torticollis) (see Chap. 40) which
is usually more irregular and sometimes increases with attempts to rotate the head
opposite to the direction of the torticollis. Essential tremor affecting the head is
nearly always associated with limb tremor, but head tremor occasionally occurs in
isolation which, in many cases, may actually be due to cervical dystonia rather than
essential tremor. Patients with Parkinson's disease much more commonly have
tremor of the jaw or lips rather than head tremor. Differential diagnosis of voice
tremor is largely limited to adductor spasmodic dysphonia which is more strained,
effortful, and staccato in type and associated with characteristic voice breaks. It is
helpful to elicit voice tremor with sustained phonation with vowel sounds such as
"ah" or "ee." Head and voice tremor are much less responsive than hand tremor to
oral medications such as beta-blockers or primidone. Botulinum toxin injections
given into the posterior cervical muscles often reduce the severity of head tremor.
By contrast, botulinum toxin vocal cord injections are usually ineffective for voice
tremor unless there is an associated component of spasmodic dysphonia.

Case

A 69-year-old woman initially presented with a 10-year history of head tremor followed several years later by mild postural tremor of her hands and voice tremor.
Treatments with propranolol, primidone, and methazolamide were unhelpful.
Botulinum toxin injections into posterior cervical muscles produced mild improvement of head tremor.

R. Bhidayasiri, D. Tarsy, *Movement Disorders: A Video Atlas*, Current Clinical Neurology,
DOI 10.1007/978-1-60327-426-5_25, © Springer Science+Business Media New York 2012

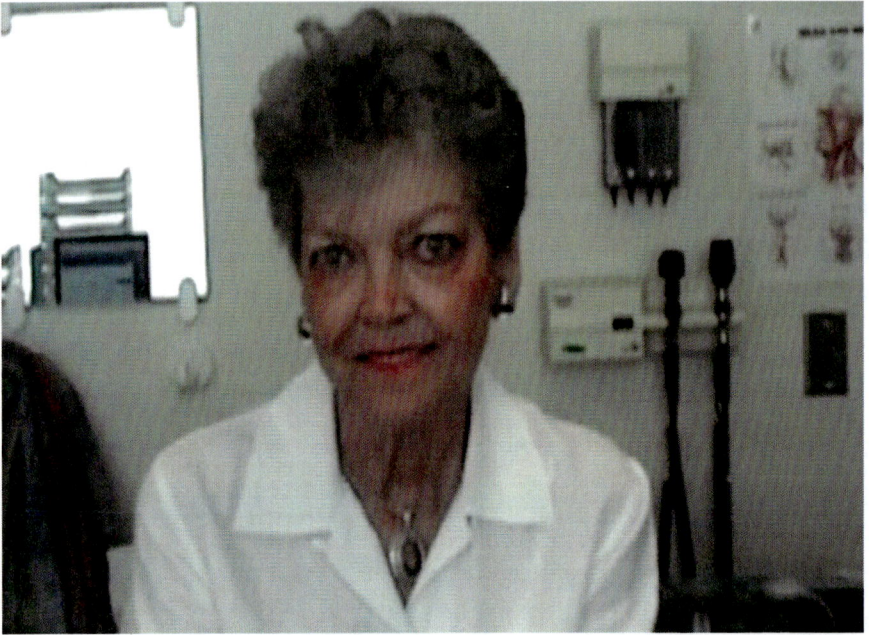

Video
The patient exhibits a mixed vertical and rotary head tremor, voice tremor, and mild finger tremor.

References

1. Louis ED, Dogu O. Isolated head tremor: part of the clinical spectrum of essential tremor? Data from population-based and clinic-based case samples. Mov Disord. 2009;24:2281–5.
2. Sulica L, Louis ED. Clinical characteristics of essential voice tremor: a study of 34 cases. Laryngoscope. 2010;120:516–28.

Chapter 26
Cerebellar Tremor

This chapter contains a video segment which can be found at the
URL: http://www.springerimages.com/Tarsy

Background

The term cerebellar tremor is often used synonymously with intention tremor.
However, several clinical types of action tremor are included in this category with
intention tremor being the most common form. Intention tremor typically increases
during the approach to a target. Action, kinetic, and titubation or stance tremors are
usually regarded as being of cerebellar origin if other signs of cerebellar dysfunction are also present. According to the consensus statement of the Movement
Disorder Society on tremor, cerebellar tremors can be diagnosed according to the
following clinical signs: (1) pure or dominant intention tremor, either unilateral or
bilateral; (2) tremor frequency usually less than 5 Hz; and (3) postural tremor present without rest tremor.

Cerebellar tremor is most commonly caused by damage to the cerebellum resulting from multiple sclerosis, stroke or hemorrhage, tumor, or certain inherited degen-
erative disorders. It may also result from chronic alcoholism or medication toxicity.
In classic cerebellar tremor, a lesion in one cerebellar hemisphere produces ipsilateral intention tremor which worsens with directed movement. Titubation is a midline truncal tremor which is a slow-frequency oscillation of the head and upper
trunk which is dependent on postural innervation due to pathology of the cerebellum and/or its afferent or efferent pathways. Effective pharmacologic treatment of
cerebellar tremor is unavailable. Deep brain stimulation surgery within the ventro-
intermediate nucleus of the thalamus has been successfully used in some forms of
intractable cerebellar tremor.

Case

A 56-year-old man with a history of alcoholic hepatitis developed increasing
difficulty with gait. He was losing control of both legs, tended to sway, and would
fall unless holding onto a railing for support. Tremor in both hands was worsening
to the point that he was unable to hold a fork, knife, or glass of water. Examination
revealed scanning speech with hypophonia. Gait was wide-based. Strength was normal but severe intention tremor was present bilaterally with inability to perform
finger-nose movements.

R. Bhidayasiri, D. Tarsy, *Movement Disorders: A Video Atlas*, Current Clinical Neurology,   54
DOI 10.1007/978-1-60327-426-5_26, © Springer Science+Business Media New York 2012

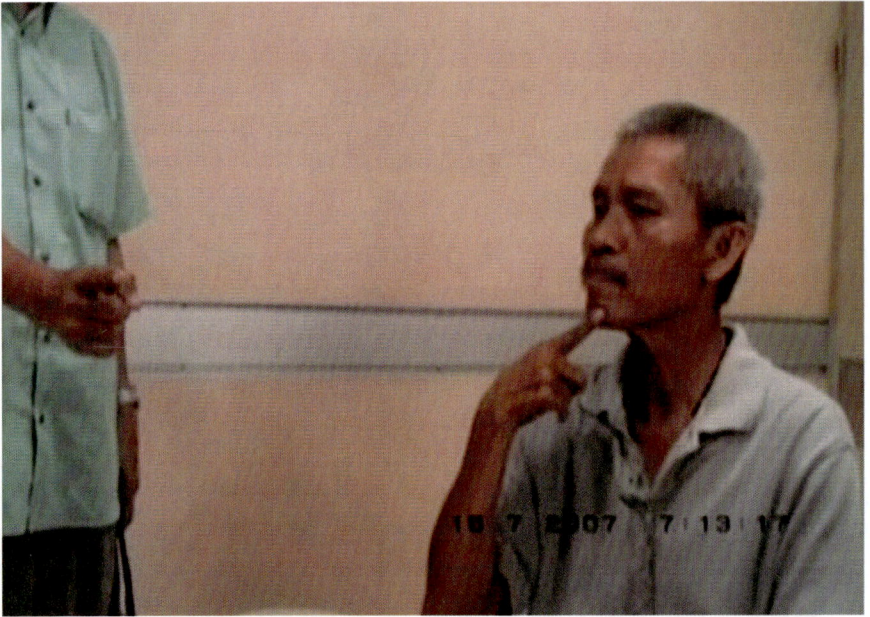

Video

The patient exhibits kinetic tremor of both upper extremities during finger-chin testing with larger amplitude limb oscillations while approaching the target of the examiner's finger. Gait is broad-based, unsteady, and requires use of a cane.

References

1. Deuschl G, Bain P, Brin M, and an Ad Hoc Scientific Committee. Consensus statement of the movement disorder society on tremor. Mov Disord. 1998;13 Suppl 3:2–23.
2. Deuschl G, Bergman H. Pathophysiology of nonparkinsonian tremor. Mov Disord. 2002;17 Suppl 3:S41–8.

Chapter 27
Holmes' Midbrain Tremor

This chapter contains a video segment which can be found at the
URL: http://www.springerimages.com/Tarsy

Background

Holmes' tremor, also known as thalamic, midbrain, or rubral tremor, is characterized by a combination of irregular resting, postural, and intention tremors of large
amplitude and slow frequency of less than 4.5 Hz. The tremor predominantly affects
the proximal upper extremities unilaterally and is often markedly activated by goal-
directed movements. Etiology is usually a structural lesion of the brainstem, cerebellum, or thalamus as a result of stroke, vascular malformation, tumor, multiple
sclerosis, trauma, or infection. There may be a variable delay of 2 weeks to 2 years
between the precipitating event and the initial appearance of tremor.

A recent study indicates that hemorrhage is the most frequent etiology of Holmes'
tremor, and the thalamus is the most commonly involved structure. The concept that
two systems, dopaminergic and the cerebellothalamic, must be involved in order to
produce Holmes' tremor has been recently challenged by a DaTSCAN study showing normal uptake of the presynaptic dopaminergic nigrostriatal system.

Case

A 21-year-old man was referred with left arm tremor that was becoming more severe
over the previous 5 months. On examination, he was alert with a reactive left pupil. The
right pupil was 7 mm and unreactive to light, and a right oculomotor palsy was present
causing impaired adduction and vertical eye movements. There was a left hemiparesis
associated with a left extensor plantar response. Severe resting, postural, and action
tremor involved the left arm. T1-weighted brain MRI showed a hypointensity in the
right paramedian midbrain consistent with a previous hemorrhage (Fig. 27.1).

References

1. Deuschl G, Bain P, Brin M, et al. Consensus statement of the Movement Disorder Society on
   tremor. Mov Disord. 1998;13 Suppl 3:2–23.
2. Gajos GA, Bogucki A, Schinwelski M, et al. The clinical and neuroimaging studies in Holmes
   tremor. Acta Neurol Scand. 2010;122:360–6.
3. Paviour DC, Jager HR, Wilkinson L, et al. Holmes' tremor: application of modern neuroimaging technique. Mov Disord. 2006;21:2260–2.

R. Bhidayasiri, D. Tarsy, *Movement Disorders: A Video Atlas*, Current Clinical Neurology,
DOI 10.1007/978-1-60327-426-5_27, © Springer Science+Business Media New York 2012

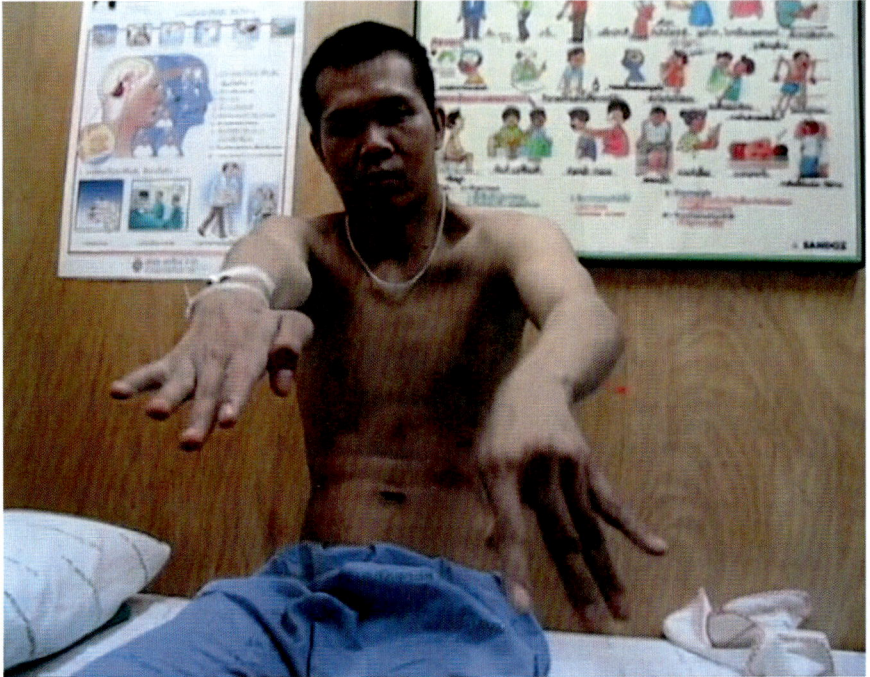

Video
Clip 1: the patient exhibits severe postural tremor of the left arm. Not shown are equally severe resting and kinetic tremor. *Clip 2*: the patient attempts goal-directed arm movements but is unable to carry them out (Video contribution from Dr. Parnsiri Chairangsaris, Pramongkutklao Hospital, Thailand).

Fig. 27.1 T1-weighted brain MRI showed a hypodensity lesion in the right paramedian midbrain.

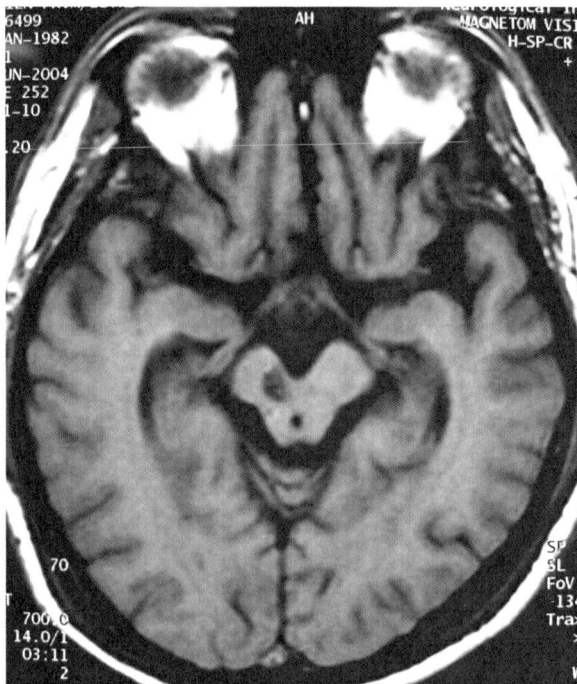

Chapter 28
Wilson's Disease with Wing-Beating Tremor

This chapter contains a video segment which can be found at the
URL: http://www.springerimages.com/Tarsy

Background

The common neurologic manifestations of Wilson's disease (WD) are dysarthria,
tremor, dystonia, parkinsonism, and gait disturbance. While all tremor types may
occur in WD, postural and resting tremors are the most common. The classical
proximal "wing-beating" tremor of WD is often missing in the early stages of the
disease. When it does appear, it is often resistant to decoppering therapy and anti-
tremor drugs and results in severe disability. Recent MRI studies indicate that WD
tremor is associated with lesions of the globus pallidus, the head of the caudate
nucleus, and the substantia nigra. There is some experience indicating that uncontrolled bilateral upper limb tremor may respond to thalamotomy.

Case

A 33-year-old man presented with a disabling tremor of both hands which had been
severe during certain actions and postures for the past year. In addition to tremor, he
had a history of jaundice, dysarthria, and behavioral disturbance. Examination
showed Kayser-Fleischer corneal rings, jaw dystonia, and postural instability with
pull testing. Tremor was severe and of the wing-beating type. Mild resting tremor of
the hands and head tremor were also present. Head tremor as well as mild resting
tremor were present. While raising his hands, an escalating tremor appeared bilaterally, particularly in the wing-beating position, which progressed into wild, flinging
movements bilaterally.

References

1. Sudmeyer M, Saleh A, Wojtecki L, et al. Wilson's disease tremor is associated with magnetic
   resonance imaging lesions in basal ganglia structures. Mov Disord. 2006;21:2134–9.
2. Bhidayasiri R. Differential diagnosis of common tremor syndromes. Postgrad Med J.
   2005;81:756–62.
3. Puschmann A, Wszolek ZK. Diagnosis and treatment of common forms of tremor. Semin
   Neurol. 2011;31:65–77.

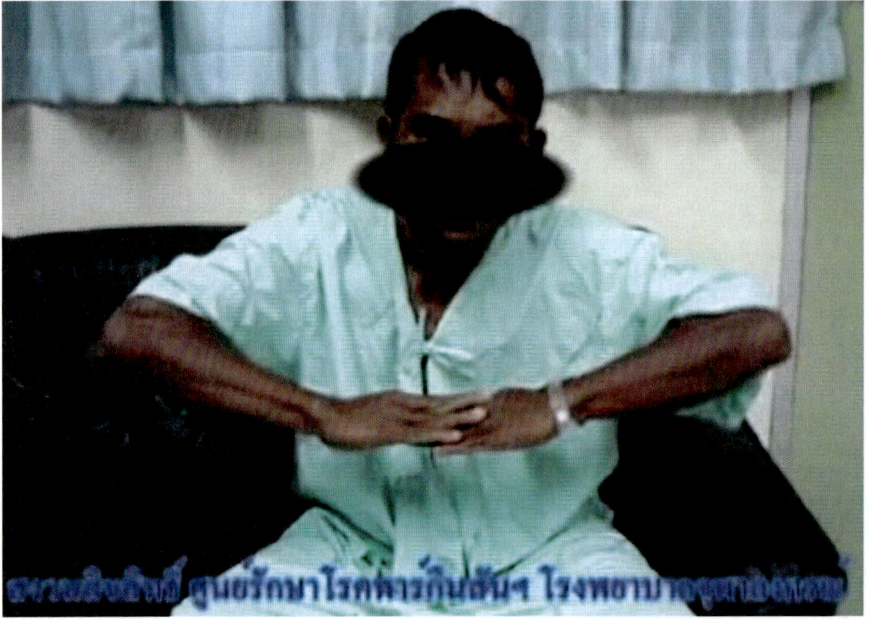

Video
The patient exhibits bilateral "wing-beating" tremor associated with mild head tremor and cervical dystonia. (Video contribution from Dr. H. Ling, Chiang Mai University Hospital, Thailand.)

Chapter 29
Primary Writing Tremor

This chapter contains a video segment which can be found at the
URL: http://www.springerimages.com/Tarsy

Background

Primary writing tremor is a relatively selective task-specific and unilateral action
tremor which occurs nearly exclusively during the act of writing. In most cases,
writing is a specific provocative factor, while in others it is provoked by pronation
of the forearm and may therefore appear during other tasks in which a similar forearm posture is adopted. Tasks in which tools are used are often affected but much
less severely than writing. It appears to be relatively nonprogressive. It has been
thought to be either a variant of essential tremor or a variant of writer's cramp with
prominent dystonic tremor. It is an alternating tremor with a usual frequency of
5–7 Hz. Similar to essential tremor, it is often improved by alcohol. Treatment is
usually unsatisfactory, but some patients have responded to primidone, propranolol,
and botulinum toxin.

Case

A 55-year-old man developed tremor of right hand while writing. Milder but similar
tremor occurred while using a screwdriver, decorating a cake, or holding a paint-
brush. It was absent while drinking from a cup, using eating utensils, shaving, or
during other motor tasks. Treatments with propranolol, primidone, trihexyphenidyl,
topiramate, gabapentin, benzodiazepines, and pregabalin were all unhelpful.

References

1. Bain PG, Findley LJ, Britton TC, et al. Primary writing tremor. Brain. 1995;118:1461–72.
2. Elble RJ, Moody C, Higgins C. Primary writing tremor. A form of focal dystonia? Mov Disord. 1990;5:118–26.
3. Rosenbaum F, Jankovic J. Focal task-specific tremor and dystonia: categorization of occupa-tional movement disorders. Neurology. 1988;38:522–7.

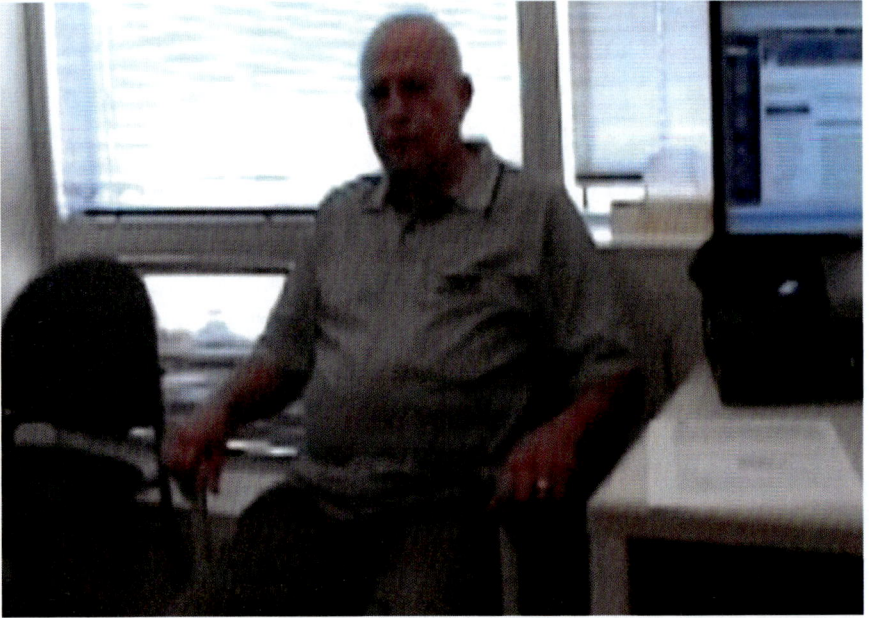

Video

Examination shows absence of tremor with arms extended or while drinking from a cup. Tremor appears immediately on beginning to write. The brief bursts of tremor which occur during writing are characteristic features of this disorder.

Chapter 30
Orthostatic Tremor

This chapter contains a video segment which can be found at the URL: http://www.springerimages.com/Tarsy

Background

Orthostatic tremor is a high frequency 14–16 Hz tremor of the legs which occurs nearly exclusively while standing and predominantly involves the lower extremities and trunk. Patients usually report unsteadiness but may also experience leg muscle cramps and have a strong need to walk, sit, or lie down to gain relief. The tremor is usually visible but is sometimes more readily palpable in the legs. The tremor may also appear with isometric contraction of upper limbs, jaw, and facial muscles. There is a high incidence of familial postural tremor among patients with orthostatic tremor, but its relationship to essential tremor is uncertain. Similar but usually lower frequency orthostatic tremor is sometimes associated with Parkinson's disease, lesions of the pons, and head trauma. Treatment with clonazepam is the initial treatment of choice but is not always effective. Other medications which have reportedly been helpful include gabapentin and levodopa.

Case

A 41-year-old woman noted onset of tremor exclusively while standing coincident with completing chemotherapy for breast cancer. The tremor persisted with slowly increasing severity for the next 8 years. She is unable to stand in lines or at social functions. Treatment with primidone and gabapentin were unhelpful while topiramate and clonazepam produced moderate relief of tremor. Examination showed a high-frequency, slightly irregular tremor in proximal muscles of both legs within several seconds of standing. Within several minutes, she began shifting her weight and was finally forced to sit in order to relieve the tremor. There was no head, voice, or arm tremor.

R. Bhidayasiri, D. Tarsy, *Movement Disorders: A Video Atlas*, Current Clinical Neurology, DOI 10.1007/978-1-60327-426-5_30, © Springer Science+Business Media New York 2012

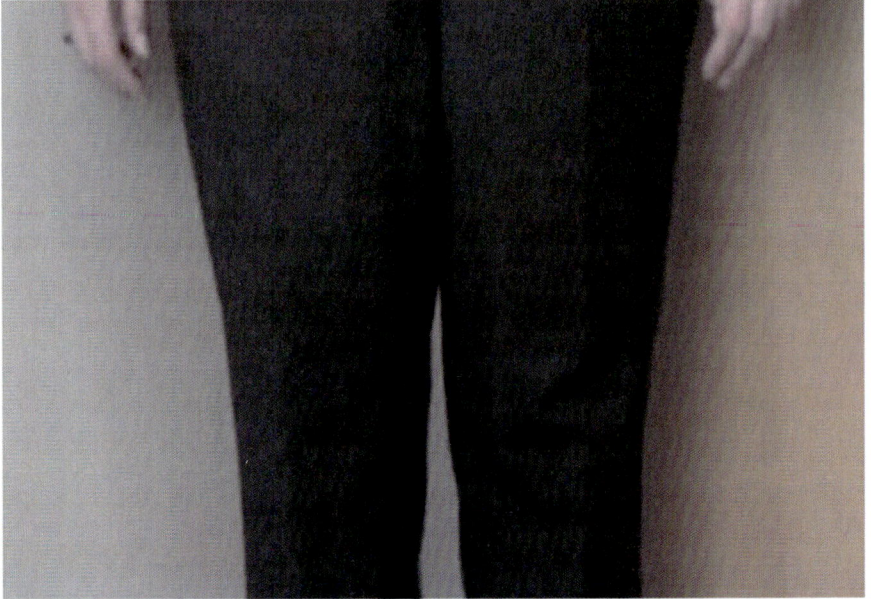

Video
The patient exhibits high-frequency, irregular tremor of her thighs while standing which disappears while walking and reappears again while standing.

References

1. Heilman KM. Orthostatic tremor. Arch Neurol. 1984;412:880–1.
2. Fitzgerald PM, Jankovic J. Orthostatic tremor: an association with essential tremor. Mov Disord. 1991;6:60–4.
3. Gabellini AS, Martinelli P, Gulli MR, et al. Orthostatic tremor: essential and symptomatic cases. Acta Neurol Scand. 1990;81:113–7.

Chapter 31
Hyperthyroid Tremor

This chapter contains a video segment which can be found at the
URL: http://www.springerimages.com/Tarsy

Background

Normal individuals have a low amplitude and high-frequency physiologic postural
tremor of the hands that is usually not visible under ordinary circumstances. There
are numerous factors which may increase the amplitude of physiologic tremor,
many of which are related to increased sympathetic activity. Drugs which increase
tremor by elevating adrenergic activity include beta-adrenergic agonists such as iso-
proterenol and epinephrine, terbutaline, amphetamines, norepinephrine reuptake
inhibitors, tricyclic antidepressants, levodopa, and xanthines such as theophylline
and caffeine. Anxiety, fright, excitement, muscle fatigue, hypoglycemia, alcohol
and opioid withdrawal, thyrotoxicosis, and pheochromocytoma also enhance adrenergic activity. There are several other drugs and toxins which increase physiologic
tremor by uncertain mechanisms such as lithium, corticosteroids, sodium valproate,
amiodarone, mercury, lead, and arsenic. Enhanced physiologic tremor is the most
common cause of postural and action tremor. Therefore, a medical rather than primary neurologic cause for tremor of this type should always be considered. Tremor
is particularly common in hyperthyroidism where it is a high-frequency and low-
amplitude tremor which resembles enhanced physiologic tremor. Its response to
propranolol suggests that it is mediated by increased adrenergic effects. Although
usually present together with other features of hyperthyroidism, tremor may sometimes be the presenting complaint.

Case

A 55-year-old nurse practitioner reported intermittent tremor of her right leg while
standing of 9 months duration, followed 2 months later by a fine postural and action
tremor of both hands occurring while suturing, drinking from a cup, and using eating utensils. She had also noticed heat intolerance, scalp hair loss, and intermittent
tachycardia. Examination showed a fine, low-amplitude, high-frequency tremor in
both hands when extended, when placed in front of her nose, and while drinking
from a cup. There were no other motor findings. Free T-4 was elevated at 4.6 and
TSH was reduced at <0.02. Thyroid scan with uptake was indicative of Graves'
disease. She was treated methimazole with control of hyperthyroidism and disap-
pearance of tremor.

R. Bhidayasiri, D. Tarsy, *Movement Disorders: A Video Atlas*, Current Clinical Neurology,   66
DOI 10.1007/978-1-60327-426-5_31, © Springer Science+Business Media New York 2012

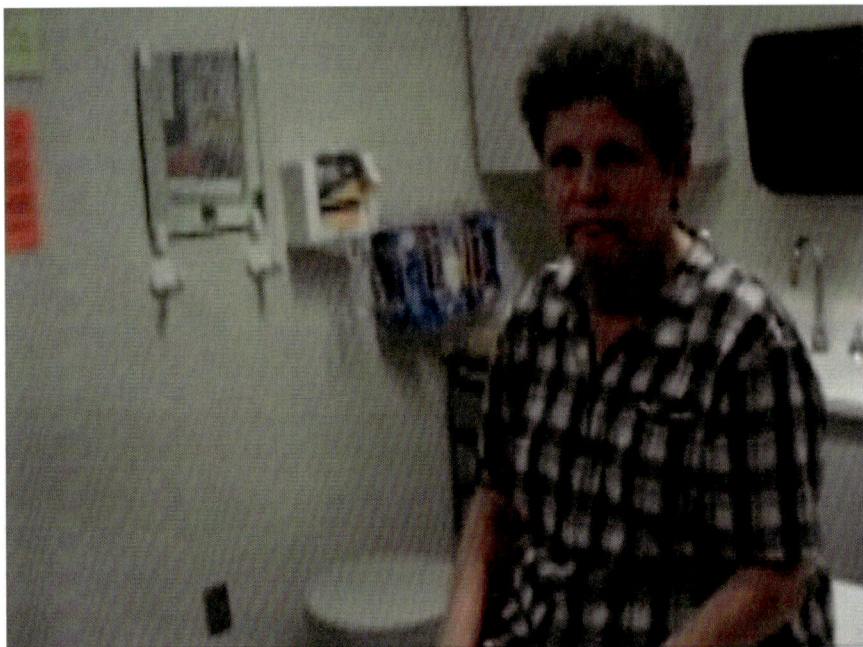

Video
The patient displays an irregular high-frequency, low-amplitude tremor of the hands involving left more than right side.

References

1. Jankovic J, Fahn S. Physiologic and pathologic tremors. Diagnosis, mechanism, and management. Ann Intern Med. 1980;93:460–5.
2. Duyff RF, den Bosch Van, Laman DM, et al. Neuromuscular findings in thyroid dysfunction: a prospective clinical and electrodiagnostic study. J Neurol Neurosurg Psychiatry. 2000;68:750–5.
3. Henderson JM, Portmann L, Van Melle G, et al. Propranolol as an adjunct therapy for hyperthyroid tremor. Eur Neurol. 1997;37:182–5.

Chapter 32
Drug-Induced Tremor

This chapter contains a video segment which can be found at the
URL: http://www.springerimages.com/Tarsy

Background

Drugs are a common cause of tremor and may produce a wide variety of tremor types
(see Chap. 31). The clinical presentation depends on the drug and possibly the predis-
positions of individual patients. There is a lengthy list of drugs which cause tremor, the
most common of which include tricyclic antidepressants, selective serotonin reuptake
inhibitors, beta-agonists, bronchodilators, corticosteroids, cyclosporine, amiodarone,
lithium, antipsychotic drugs, metoclopramide, nicotine, and valproic acid.

A tremor may be considered to be drug-induced if it occurs within a reasonable
time frame following drug ingestion. A careful history should be obtained to exclude
tremors which may have been present before drug initiation. Differentiation of
drug-induced tremor from other causes requires a thorough history and physical
examination. Important considerations include exclusion of other medical causes
such as hyperthyroidism, a temporal relationship between the drug exposure and
onset of tremor, a dose-response relationship between dose and tremor severity, and
symmetrical involvement.

Case

A 45-year-old woman with a long history of bipolar disorder presented to an outpatient
psychiatric clinic because of progressive tremor for the past 3 months. She had been on
lithium for at least 5 years and a lithium level 6 months previously was in therapeutic
range. Because of worsening depression, her physician had prescribed paroxetine
3 months earlier. Examination revealed bilateral resting and action tremor, affecting
both bilateral upper extremities. The tremor made her unable to perform daily tasks
such as writing and drinking from a glass without spilling. The tremor dramatically
improved when paroxetine was discontinued while lithium was left unchanged.

References

1. Morgan JC, Sethi KD. Drug-induced tremors. Lancet Neurol. 2005;4:866–76.
2. Factor SA. Lithium-induced movement disorders. In: Sethi KD, editor. Drug-induced movement disorders. New York: Marcel Dekker; 2004. p. 209–31.
3. Tarsy D. Miscellaneous drug-induced movement disorders. In: Factor S, Lang AE, Weiner WJ,
   editors. Drug-induced movement disorders. Malden: Blackwell Futura; 2005. p. 430–1.

R. Bhidayasiri, D. Tarsy, *Movement Disorders: A Video Atlas*, Current Clinical Neurology,   68
DOI 10.1007/978-1-60327-426-5_32, © Springer Science+Business Media New York 2012

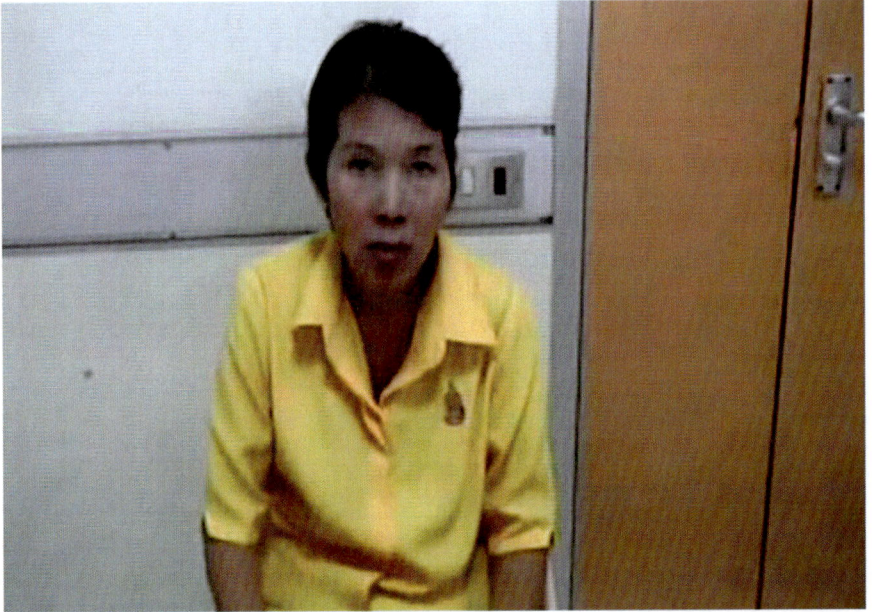

Video
This patient, who is taking lithium and paroxetine, exhibits a high-frequency, low-amplitude tremor at rest, a postural tremor with arms extended, and action tremor involving both hands symmetrically. There is no asterixis. The tremor is absent while walking.

Chapter 33
Dystonic Tremor

This chapter contains a video segment which can be found at the
URL: http://www.springerimages.com/Tarsy

Background

Dystonic tremor refers to the presence of tremor in a body part which is also affected
by dystonia. Dystonic tremor is usually irregular, focal, variable in amplitude, and
relatively low in frequency (usually less than 7 Hz). When it affects the limbs, dystonic tremor is usually a postural and/or kinetic tremor which is usually absent at
rest. A common example of dystonic tremor is the irregular and jerky head tremor
which often accompanies cervical dystonia (see Chap. 40). The precise relationship
of dystonic tremor to dystonia has been debated. Dystonic movements may be
inherently tremulous in nature due to co-contraction of agonist and antagonist muscles. In some cases, such as in cervical dystonia, dystonic tremor may result from
conscious or unconscious attempts by the patient to restore body posture toward
normal. According to the consensus statement of the Movement Disorder Society
on tremor, dystonic tremor differs from a tremor which is simply associated with
dystonia. The latter refers to the presence of tremor in a body part unaffected by the
patient's dystonia.

Case

A 45-year-old woman presented with 5-year history of head deviation associated
with jerky head movements. Examination revealed a complex cervical dystonia
associated with jerky head movements. Elevation of the right shoulder elevation
was also present. Head tremor and dystonia both partially improved after treatment
with botulinum toxin.

References

1. Deuschl G, Bain P, Brin M, et al. Consensus statement of the Movement Disorder Society on
   tremor. Mov Disord. 1998;13 Suppl 3:2–23.
2. Deuschl G, Heinen F, Kleedorfer B, et al. Clinical and polymyographic investigation of spasmodic torticollis. J Neurol. 1992;239:9–15.

R. Bhidayasiri, D. Tarsy, *Movement Disorders: A Video Atlas*, Current Clinical Neurology,   70
DOI 10.1007/978-1-60327-426-5_33, © Springer Science+Business Media New York 2012

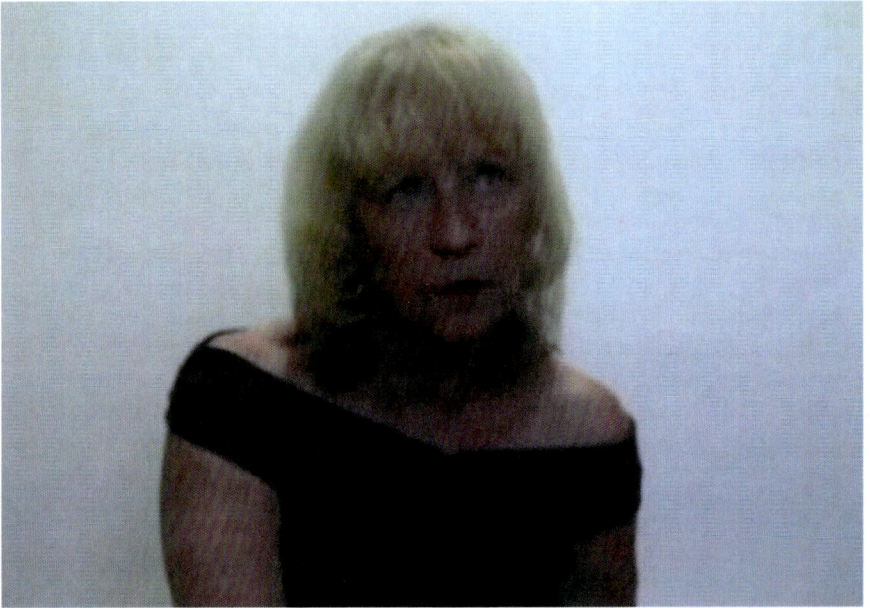

Video
Clip 1: the patient exhibits a complex cervical dystonia producing left rotational torticollis, right laterocollis, and right shoulder elevation. The dystonic head posture is associated with mixed vertical ("yes-yes") and horizontal ("no-no") tremulous and jerky head movements. *Clip 2*: another patient displays a continuous jerky postural and rest tremor in right upper extremity in a variety of positions. The tremor appeared in early childhood on a background of perinatal distress and forceps delivery. Botulinum toxin has shown partial improvement in the tremor.

Chapter 34
Neuropathic Tremor

This chapter contains a video segment which can be found at the
URL: http://www.springerimages.com/Tarsy

Background

Neuropathic tremor is assumed to be present if a patient develops tremor together
with a peripheral neuropathy in the absence of any other neurological disorder.
Certain peripheral neuropathies tend to produce tremor more often than others, particularly demyelinating polyneuropathies. These tremors are usually postural and
kinetic with frequencies of 3–6 Hz in arm and hand muscles. The frequency in hand
muscles can be lower than in proximal arm muscles in patients with gammopathies.
Fortunately, most of these patients have only a slight tremor. No specific drugs are
available for this disorder, but in most cases, it is are not severe enough to require
pharmacological treatment. The pathophysiology of neuropathic tremor is thought
to result from an interaction of peripheral and central nervous system factors.
However, the major peripheral abnormality appears to be slowing of peripheral
nerve conduction velocity and a resultant distortion of afferent signals.

Case

A 43-year-old Thai monk with a long history of undiagnosed peripheral neuropathy
presented with a 3-year history of tremor in both hands. His main complaint was
weakness in his hands which was attributed to neuropathy and a certain degree of
cervical radiculopathy. Because of hand weakness, he found that the tremor made
hand functioning more difficult in daily tasks such as holding a cup of water or eating utensils. Examination revealed no rest tremor. He had a left wrist drop. There
was also wasting and weakness of the intrinsic hand muscles. A low-frequency
postural tremor was present bilaterally.

References

1. Bain PG, Britton TC, Jenkins IH, et al. Tremor associated with benign IgM paraproteinemic
neuropathy. Brain. 1996;119:789–99.
2. Deuschl G, Bergman H. Pathophysiology of nonparkinsonian tremors. Mov Disord. 2002;17
Suppl 3:S41–8.

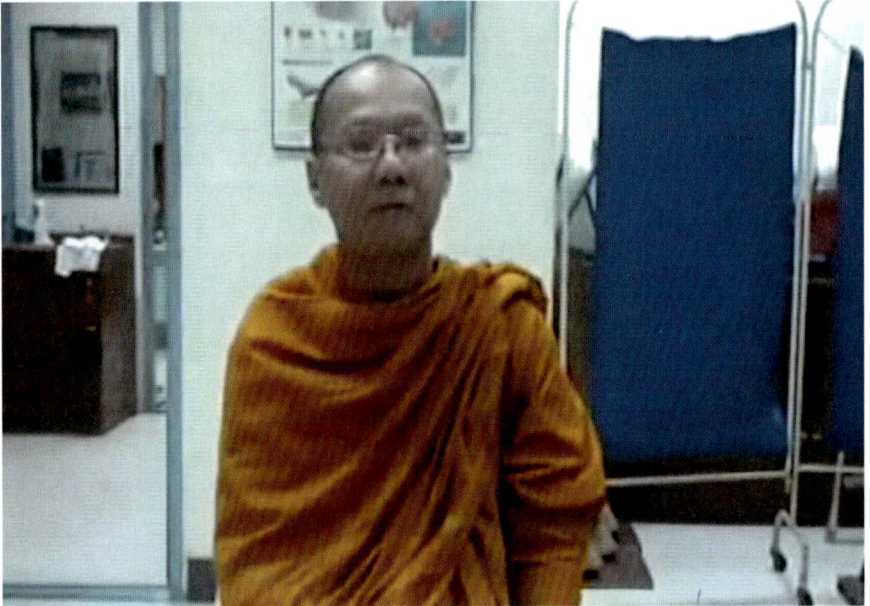

Video
The patient has a left wrist drop. There is weakness of the intrinsic hand muscles bilaterally. No resting tremor is present, but bilateral distal postural and action tremor is present which is greater on the right than left side.

Chapter 35
Psychogenic Tremor

This chapter contains a video segment which can be found at the
URL: http://www.springerimages.com/Tarsy

Background

Psychogenic tremor is probably the most common of the psychogenic movement
disorders and may have different clinical presentations. The following clinical features suggest psychogenic tremor: (1) sudden onset and/or remission of the tremor;
(2) unusual combinations of rest, postural, and action tremors; (3) reduced tremor
frequency and amplitude when distracted, such as when asked to carry out repetitive
voluntary movements of the contralateral hand; (4) entrainment of tremor frequency
to match the frequency of a repetitive task performed in another limb; (5) previous
history of somatization; and (6) the appearance of other unexplained neurologic
signs. Almost 75% of presenting patients are female. Commonly there are preceding precipitating events such as work-related injuries or emotional trauma. Other
useful clues are hand tremor without finger tremor and an associated artificial
appearing and an effortful slowness of voluntary movements. Most patients present
with unilateral tremor affecting the wrist, elbow, or shoulder, which is unlike PD
tremor which usually begins more distally in the fingers. Comorbidity with psychiatric disorders is common including somatoform disorders such as pain, diffuse
sensory loss, conversion disorder, and depression. About 20% of patients are
involved in litigation or compensation issues.

The diagnosis of psychogenic tremor is not only a diagnosis of exclusion but
should be a positive diagnosis based on history, clinical signs, and investigations. A
multifaceted approach including neuropsychiatric evaluation and psychotherapy
should be considered. Prognosis for recovery is typically poor if the condition persists for more than a year.

Case

A 45-year-old woman presented with the sudden onset of right hand tremor following a motor vehicle accident. She stated the accident caused intense pain in her right
shoulder followed immediately by onset of tremor. In addition, she complained that
her vision was blurred, that she stuttered when speaking, and that her gait was
unsteady. Examination revealed tremor with variable frequencies in her right hand
which was present both at rest and during action. Entrainment occurred while carrying out repetitive movements of her right hand.

R. Bhidayasiri, D. Tarsy, *Movement Disorders: A Video Atlas*, Current Clinical Neurology,
DOI 10.1007/978-1-60327-426-5_35, © Springer Science+Business Media New York 2012

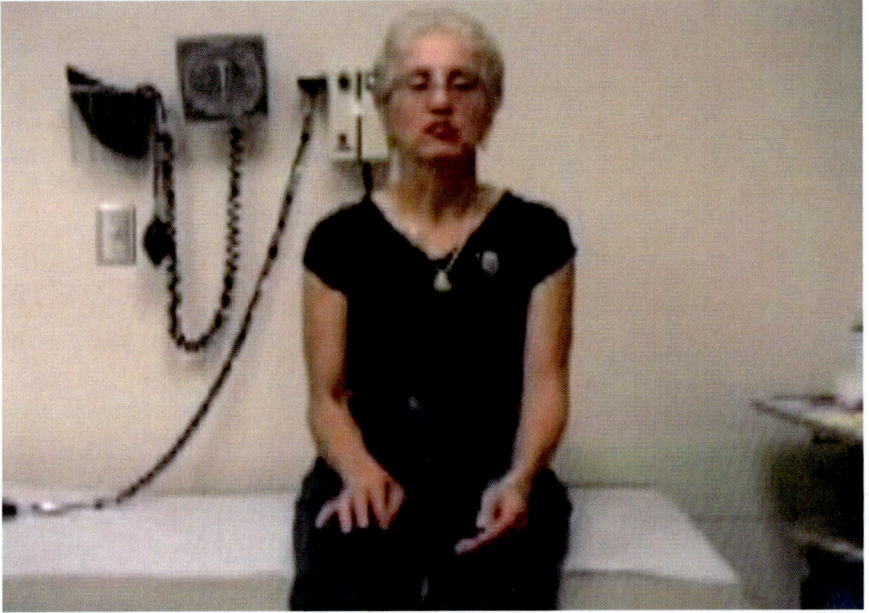

Video

The patient exhibits an irregular, large amplitude tremor of her right hand and fingers which is present at rest, in various postures, and during action. Tremor amplitude and frequency are variable. Sometimes the tremor ceases spontaneously and while she is being distracted with other motor tasks. Tremor entrainment occurs when she is asked to open and close her opposite hand.

References

1. Deuschl G, Bain P, Brin M, an Ad Hoc Scientific Committee. Consensus statement of the Movement Disorder Society on tremor. Mov Disord. 1998;13 Suppl 3:2–23.
2. Miyasaki JI, Sa DS, Galvez-Jimenez N, et al. Psychogenic movement disorders. Can J Neurol Sci. 2003;30 Suppl 1:S94–100.
3. McKeon A, Ahlskog JE, Bower JH, et al. Psychogenic tremor: long-term prognosis in patients with electrophysiologically-confirmed disease. Mov Disord. 2009;24:72–6.
4. Espay AJ, Goldenhar LM, Voon V, et al. Opinions and clinical practices related to diagnosing and managing patients with psychogenic movement disorders: an international survey of Movement Disorder Society members. Mov Disord. 2009;24:1366–74.

Part III
Dystonia

Chapter 36
Examination of a Patient with Non-DYT1 Generalized Dystonia

This chapter contains a video segment which can be found at the
URL: http://www.springerimages.com/Tarsy

Background

The term "dystonia" was originally coined to name a disorder causing variable muscle tone and recurrent muscle spasm. What is now called primary dystonia was initially called dystonia musculorum deformans and later primary torsion dystonia (PTD). Dystonia causes sustained muscle contractions, repetitive twisting movements, and abnormal postures of the trunk, neck, face, or extremities. Dystonia results from involuntary co-contraction of agonist and antagonist muscles with overflow of muscle contractions into adjacent muscles. Dystonic movements can be either slow or rapid, change during different activities or postures, and may become fixed in advanced cases. Except for occasional tremor or myoclonus, the rest of the neurological examination is normal. Primary generalized dystonia is a progressive and potentially very disabling disorder which begins in childhood or adolescence and is linked to several genetic loci. Many cases are autosomal dominant caused by a guanine-adenine-guanine (GAG) deletion in the *DYT1* gene, resulting in a glutamate deletion in torsin A, a brain protein of uncertain function. This gene defect accounts for 80% of early onset cases in Ashkenazi Jewish individuals and up to 50% of cases in non-Jewish individuals. Penetrance is about 30% and clinical expression varies from generalized dystonia to occasional adult-onset limb dystonias. It begins as a focal action dystonia, usually of one foot, before age 26 with most cases beginning in childhood. Childhood-onset cases commonly evolve to generalized dystonia which produces a major disfiguring disability due to severe gait and posture abnormalities. Medical treatment is limited to high-dose anticholinergic drugs such as trihexyphenidyl or benztropine, tetrabenazine, and oral or intrathecal baclofen. Globus pallidus deep brain stimulation (DBS) is the most effective treatment for PTD. Non-*DYT1* generalized dystonia is phenotypically similar or even identical to *DYT1* generalized dystonia.

Case

A 14-year-old boy presented with non-*DYT1* generalized dystonia which began with abnormal posturing of his left leg at age 2 and progressed to include involuntary movements of his upper limbs and neck by age 4. Increased gait disorder evolved over several years with inability to walk independently by age 8. He remained able to walk on his knees or crawl. Progressive dysarthria without dysphagia associated with facial and lingual dystonia began during the past year. Examination showed dystonic posturing of his legs which crossed over each other causing inability to walk but allowing him to crawl on his knees. There was distal more than proximal dystonic posturing of his arms and lower facial and lingual dystonia with marked dysarthria. The rest of his neurological examination was normal. Brain MRI, *DYT1* testing, and numerous metabolic tests for causes of childhood-onset dystonia were negative. Earlier in the course, trihexyphenidyl produced temporary benefit. Globus pallidus DBS was ineffective in reversing the dystonia.

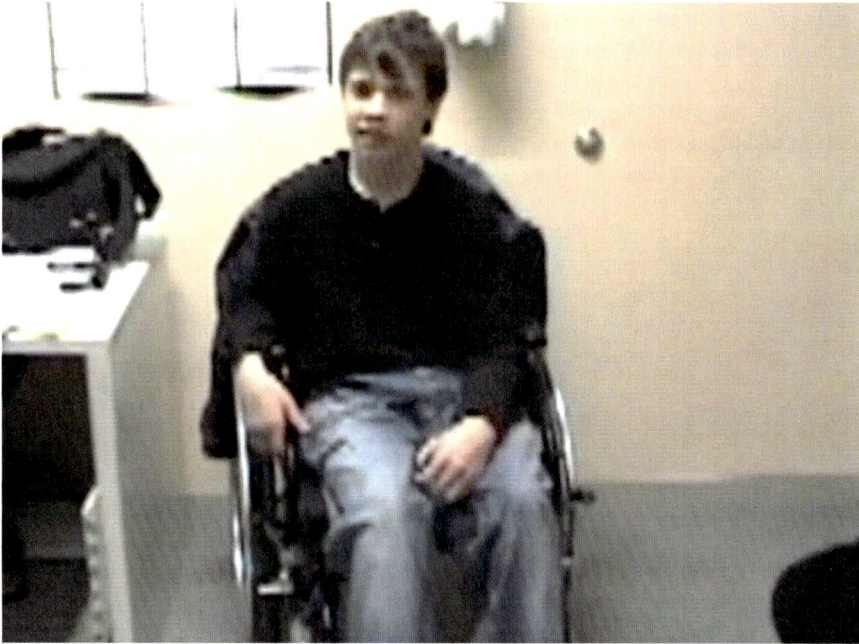

Video
The patient is being examined. He displays dystonic posturing of both hands, adduction postures of the legs, action-induced inversion and plantarflexion of the right foot while walking on his knees, occasional myoclonic jerks of the right arm and leg, and dystonic speech.

References

1. Tarsy D, Simon DK. Dystonia. N Engl J Med. 2006;355:818–29.
2. Bhidayasiri R, Tarsy D. Treatment of dystonia. Expert Rev Neurother. 2006;6:863–86.
3. Muller U. The monogenic primary dystonias. Brain. 2009;132:2005–25.

Chapter 37
DYT1 Generalized Dystonia

This chapter contains a video segment which can be found at the
URL: http://www.springerimages.com/Tarsy

Background

DYT1 or Oppenheim's dystonia is recognized as the most common form of early onset
primary dystonia. It accounts for 16–53% of early onset dystonia in non-Jewish popu-
lations but can be as high as 80–90% among Ashkenazi Jews. Typically, *DYT1* dystonia begins in early childhood with a focal action dystonia involving the lower more
commonly than the upper limb. Lower limb dystonia typically causes unilateral foot
inversion and plantar-flexion postures while walking. In early stages, patients are
often able to run or dance without exhibiting foot dystonia. Dystonia then gradually
spreads to involve other body regions, becomes less-action specific, and becomes
increasingly present at rest. Patients presenting with lower limb dystonia have a relatively poor prognosis with a greater likelihood of becoming generalized. By contrast,
children presenting at an older age, often in adolescence, with upper limb or cranio-
cervical dystonia are less likely to develop generalized dystonia.

    DYT1 dystonia is caused by a CAG deletion in the coding region of the *TOR1A*
gene. TorsinA is a member of a superfamily of ATPases which is believed to be
involved in cellular trafficking of dopamine transporters and other membrane-bound
proteins. The *DYT1* mutation is transmitted with autosomal dominant inheritance
with a penetrance of about 30%. A genetic test is commercially available and is
recommended for patients with onset of any form of dystonia before age 26 and/or
a family history of early onset dystonia. Children with *DYT1* dystonia often respond
to high doses of anticholinergic drugs. Botulinum toxin may be used for selected
focal manifestations. Treatment of *DYT1* dystonia and other forms of childhood
onset generalized dystonia has improved considerably since the introduction of surgical pallidotomy and pallidal deep brain stimulation.

Case

A 9-year-old Ashkenazi Jewish boy was brought by his mother due to a decline in
physical performance. He used to be a top runner but later experienced left ankle
pain while running. There was no family history of dystonia. On examination, there
was no dystonia at rest. Mild right arm dystonia was observed when he extended
both arms. There was mild bilateral foot inversion while walking which was worse
on the left side. Foot inversion became more obvious when he ran causing pain in
his left ankle. He sometimes fell when attempting to stop running.

R. Bhidayasiri, D. Tarsy, *Movement Disorders: A Video Atlas*, Current Clinical Neurology,
DOI 10.1007/978-1-60327-426-5_37, © Springer Science+Business Media New York 2012

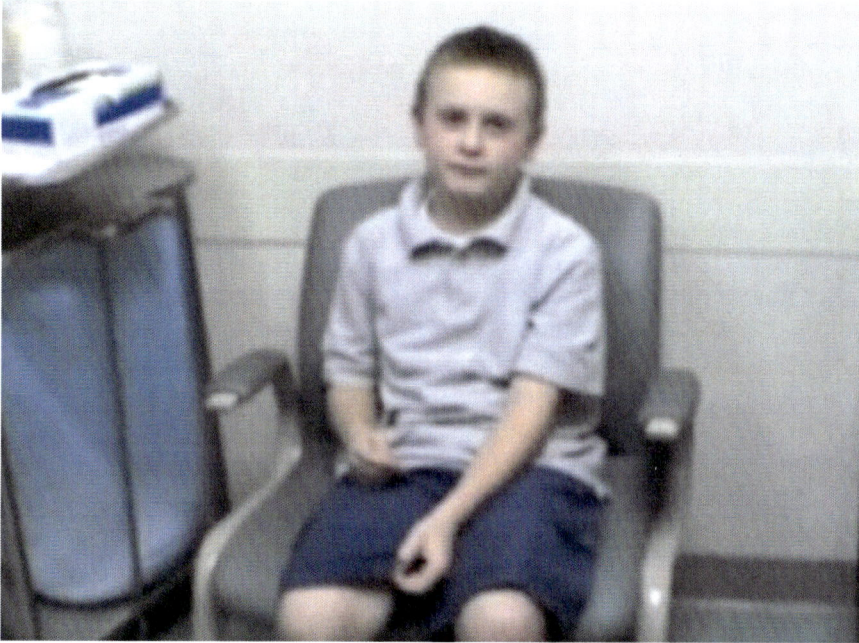

Video

Clip 1: the patient exhibits mild bilateral foot dystonia. While walking, this gives the appearance of a mild left footdrop, while on the right side he lands with his foot on its outer aspect with extensor posturing of the large toe. Later in the video, he sits with his left foot inverted. While standing, the right foot and toes are plantarflexed while the left foot is inverted. *Clip 2*: another *DYT1* patient developed cervical and axial dystonia for the first time at age 18. His trunk is flexed at the waist, hyperextended in the lower thoracic region, tilted to the right, and concave to the left in a typical "dromedary" posture. There is also cervical dystonia with a mixture of retrocollis, laterocollis, and rotational torticollis. While walking, he uses a "sensory trick" of holding his left hand to the back of his head to stabilize his posture.

References

1. Ozelius LJ, Kramer PL, Moskowitz CB, et al. Human gene for torsion dystonia located on chromosome 9q32-q34. Neuron. 1989;2:1427–34.
2. Bhidayasiri R, Pulst S-M. Dystonia (*DYT*) genetic loci. Eur J Paediatr Neurol. 2005;9:367–70.
3. Bressman SB, De Leon D, Kramer PL, et al. Dystonia in Ashkenazi Jews: clinical characterization of a founder mutation. Ann Neurol. 1994;36:771–7.

Chapter 38
Segmental Dystonia Treated with Deep Brain Stimulation

This chapter contains a video segment which can be found at the URL: http://www.springerimages.com/Tarsy

Background

Dystonia causes sustained muscle contractions, repetitive twisting movements, and abnormal postures of the trunk, neck, face, or extremities (see Chap. 36). Dystonic movements can be either slow or rapid, change during different activities or postures, and may become fixed in advanced cases. Except for occasional tremor or myoclonus, the rest of the neurological examination is normal. Childhood onset generalized dystonia typically begins as a focal action dystonia, usually of one foot, and progresses over several years to become generalized (see Chap. 37). Cases presenting in adolescence more commonly begin in one upper extremity or in the cervical-thoracic region and are more slowly progressive (see Chap. 37). Adult-onset primary dystonia usually involves cervical, cranial, or upper limb muscles but sometimes presents with segmental distribution and rarely becomes generalized. High-dose anticholinergic drugs such as trihexyphenidyl or benztropine are less well tolerated in adults than in children. Globus pallidus deep brain stimulation (DBS) is worth consideration in adult onset segmental dystonia.

Case

A 57-year-old man had onset of writer's cramp 17 years previously. Six years previously, he had the abrupt onset of cervical dystonia with rotational torticollis to the left side. A large number of medications were unhelpful including trihexyphenidyl, diazepam, clonazepam, reserpine, haloperidol, Clozaril, baclofen, and valproate. Examination showed repetitive, forceful spasmodic head jerks to the left side and backward which were stabilized by leaning his head against a wall or placing one hand on his face. There was mild perioral dyskinesia and excessive hand grip while writing. There was right-sided lateral tilt of his trunk and jerky dystonic movements of his arms while walking. Several rounds of botulinum toxin injections were administered for cervical dystonia with minimal benefit. Bilateral globus pallidus (GPi) deep brain stimulation was carried out within 2 years of his presentation which produced marked relief of axial and upper extremity dystonia but only modest control of his spasmodic cervical dystonia.

R. Bhidayasiri, D. Tarsy, *Movement Disorders: A Video Atlas*, Current Clinical Neurology, DOI 10.1007/978-1-60327-426-5_38, © Springer Science+Business Media New York 2012

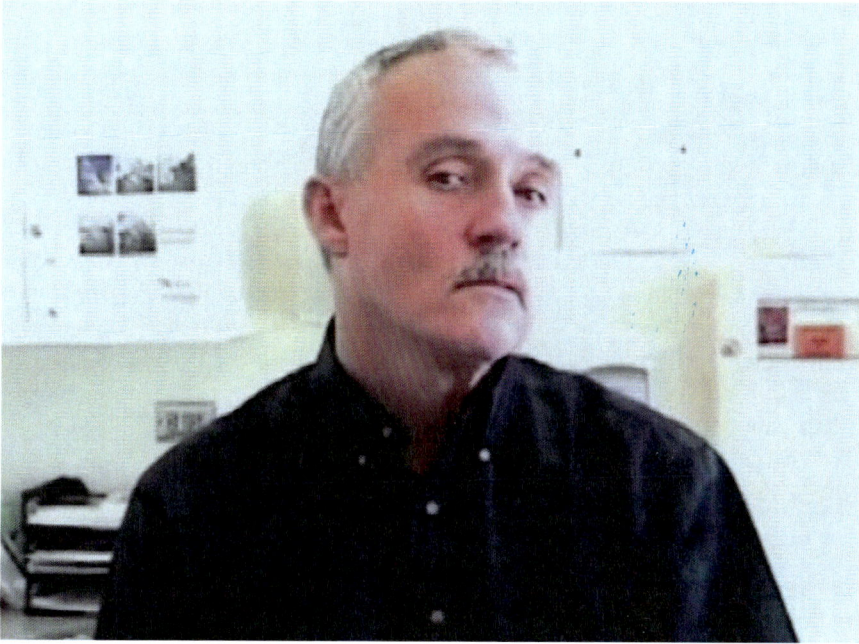

Video

Clip 1: while seated, the patient exhibits recurrent spasmodic left rotational torticollis and retrocollis together with adduction and extension posturing of his upper extremities. While walking, he exhibits jerky right lateral deviation of his upper trunk, recurrent jerky flexion at his right elbow, hyperextension and internal rotation of his left arm, and abortive attempts to stabilize his head with his hand. While writing, he exhibits perioral dystonia, repeated elevation of his right arm, slow writing, and mild spasmodic rotational torticollis to the left side. *Clip 2*: following GPi-DBS, while seated he displays less severe rotational torticollis and retrocollis with absence of upper limb dystonia. While walking, he displays right rotational torticollis without trunk or limb dystonia. He now writes faster and more easily without elevation of his right arm.

References

1. Bressman SB, Sabatti C, Raymond D, et al. The *DYT1* phenotype and guidelines for diagnostic testing. Neurology. 2000;54:1746–52.
2. Fasano A, Nardocci N, Emanuele E, et al. Non-*DYT1* early-onset primary torsion dystonia: comparison with *DYT1* phenotype and review of the literature. Mov Disord. 2006;21:1411–8.
3. Kupsch A, Benecke R, Muller J, et al. Pallidal deep brain stimulation in primary generalized or segmental dystonia. N Engl J Med. 2006;355:1978–90.

Chapter 39
Cervical Dystonia: Rotational Torticollis

This chapter contains a video segment which can be found at the
URL: http://www.springerimages.com/Tarsy

Background

Cervical dystonia (CD), also known as spasmodic torticollis, produces several varieties of abnormal head posture. The most common of these is rotational torticollis. In many patients, there is an associated laterocollis, usually to the side opposite the rotation, which creates the image of "a robin looking at the worm." In some cases, the laterocollis may be ipsilateral to the side of rotation. The second most common abnormality of head posture is laterocollis which is typically associated with shoulder elevation ipsilateral to the direction of head tilt. Pure retrocollis and anterocollis are less common forms of CD and more often occur in combination with rotational torticollis or laterocollis. Most individuals with CD have some combination of these abnormal postures. When sustained, the abnormal posture is referred to as tonic, while "spasmodic" torticollis is associated with jerky head movements or a more rhythmic dystonic head tremor (see Chap. 40). Neck and/or shoulder pain is present in 75% of patients with CD and is often the patient's chief complaint. Sensory "tricks" such as placing a finger or hand on the chin or cheek are often used to correct the abnormal posture. CD is the most common adult onset focal dystonia. Women are affected more commonly than men, and mean age of onset is in the fifth decade. Once established, there is little progression in the severity of CD, although segmental involvement of the arm or shoulder sometimes occurs. Several families with genetically determined forms of CD, usually occurring in combination with other segmental dystonias such as *DYT 6*, *DYT 7*, and *DYT 13* have been identified. Differential diagnosis includes secondary forms of torticollis caused by congenital or acquired disorders of the cervical spine, cervical disc disease, and tumors of the posterior fossa, foramen magnum, and cervical spinal cord. In many cases, patients with essential tremor limited to the head are in fact suffering from dystonic head tremor due to CD with mild abnormality of head posture. Botulinum toxin is the most effective treatment for CD. Anticholinergic drugs usually produce little or only partial benefit, while benzodiazepines may be helpful for relief of pain. Posterior ramicectomy is less commonly used now than in the past while favorable experience with deep brain stimulation of the globus pallidus has begun to accumulate.

R. Bhidayasiri, D. Tarsy, *Movement Disorders: A Video Atlas*, Current Clinical Neurology, DOI 10.1007/978-1-60327-426-5_39, © Springer Science+Business Media New York 2012

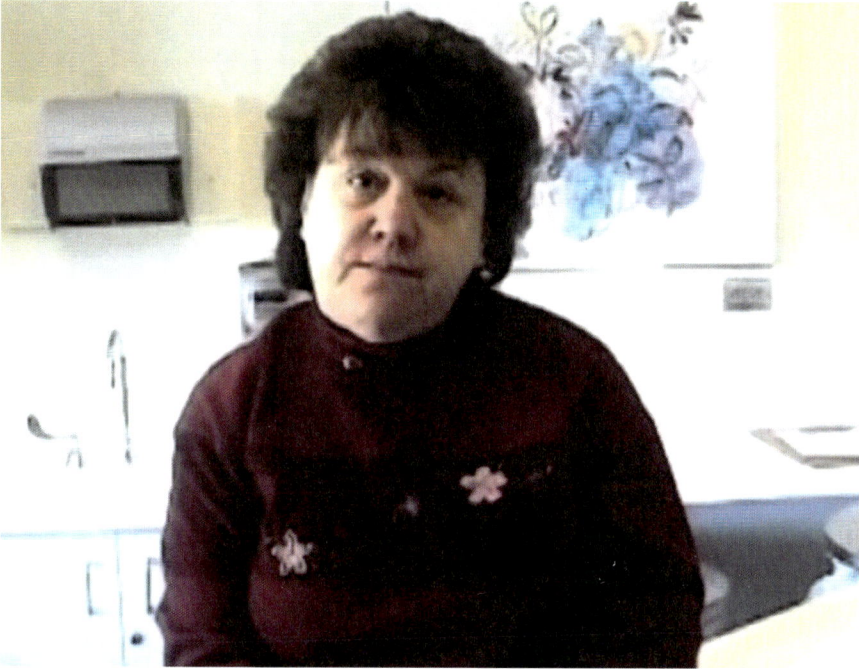

Video

The patient displays extreme tonic rotation of her head to the left side. She is able to rotate it nearly fully to the opposite side. With her head in midline position, mild left laterocollis with left shoulder elevation is also evident.

Case

A 56-year-old woman presented with involuntary rotation of her head to the left of a year's duration with increasingly limited ability to turn her head to the right side. Placing her hand against her neck or shoulder on the left side partially alleviated the movements. She has been successfully treated with botulinum toxin type A for 14 years.

References

1. Chan J, Brin MF, Fahn S. Idiopathic cervical dystonia: clinical characteristics. Mov Disord. 1991;6:119–26.
2. Jankovic J, Leder S, Warner D, Schwartz K. Cervical dystonia: clinical findings and associated movement disorders. Neurology. 1991;41:1088–91.
3. Tarsy D, First ER. Painful cervical dystonia: clinical features and response to treatment with botulinum toxin. Mov Disord. 1999;14:1043–5.

Chapter 40
Cervical Dystonia: Torticollis with Dystonic Head Tremor

This chapter contains a video segment which can be found at the
URL: http://www.springerimages.com/Tarsy

Background

Cervical dystonia (CD) is often associated with dystonic head tremor. In some cases, the head tremor is much more apparent than the abnormal head posture which may be relatively subtle. Differential diagnosis includes titubation and essential tremor limited to the head and neck. Titubation occurs as a component of midline cerebellar ataxia and is accompanied by cerebellar findings. Essential tremor affecting the head is more jerky and irregular than dystonic tremor, rarely occurs in isolation, and is nearly always associated with postural or action tremor of the upper extremities or voice tremor (see Chap. 25). Dystonic head tremor is often but not always more prominent when the patient attempts to turn the head away from the abnormal head posture. Treatment with botulinum toxin injections into the posterior cervical muscles bilaterally is usually effective in reducing the amplitude of dystonic head tremor.

Case

A 47-year-old man experienced head tremor for 10 years with only slight hand tremor. A diagnosis of essential tremor was made by several neurologists but medications for essential tremor were unhelpful. Examination showed mild tonic rotational torticollis to the left side together with horizontal head tremor. Electromyography showed a pattern of continuous spasm with tremor in splenius and semispinalis muscles bilaterally. Botulinum toxin injections into these muscles partially alleviated both the torticollis and head tremor.

References

1. Chan J, Brin M, Fahn S. Idiopathic cervical dystonia: clinical characteristics. Mov Disord. 1991;6:119–26.
2. Jankovic J, Leder S, Warner D, et al. Cervical dystonia: clinical findings and associated movement disorders. Neurology. 1991;41:1088–91.
3. Dauer WT, Burke RE, Greene P, Fahn S. Current concepts on the clinical features, aetiology and management of idiopathic cervical dystonia. Brain. 1998;121:547–60.

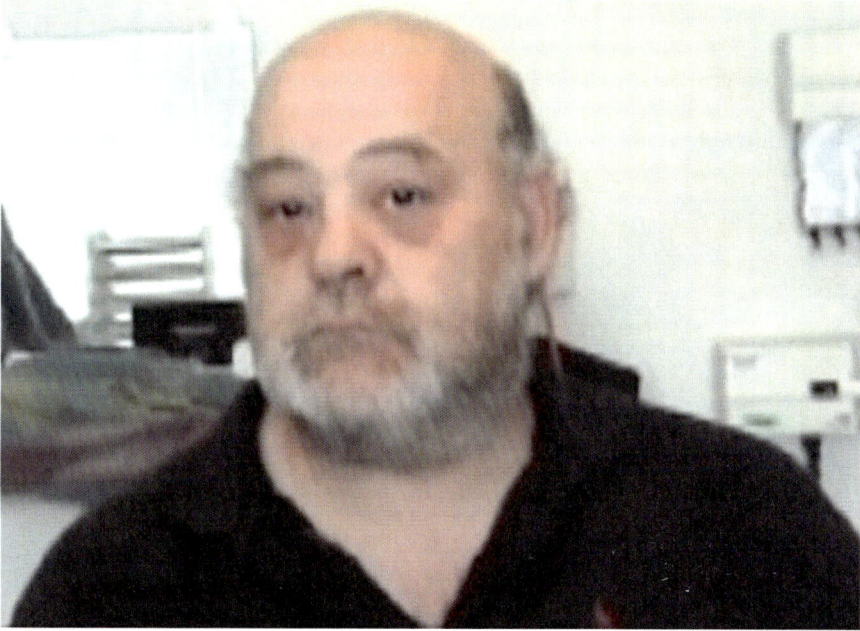

Video

At rest, the patient exhibits 25° of right-sided rotation with continuous, irregular horizontal head tremor. Rotational range of motion is full. There is no postural tremor in the upper extremities.

Chapter 41
Cervical Dystonia: Anterocollis

This chapter contains a video segment which can be found at the
URL: http://www.springerimages.com/Tarsy

Background

Anterocollis usually accompanies other forms of cervical dystonia such as rotational torticollis or laterocollis but may occur in isolation. Pure anterocollis sometimes occurs as a dystonic manifestation of multiple system atrophy. Anterocollis
must be differentiated from "dropped head syndrome" in which a myopathy of the
paraspinal extensor muscles is present which causes weakness of neck extension.

Case

A 48-year-old woman with a history of mild torticollis, reportedly present since age
14, presented with increasing symptoms including a combination of left-sided torticollis and laterocollis with shoulder elevation and head tremor. Several years later,
she developed a component of anterocollis down and to the left side. She was successfully treated with botulinum toxin A for the next 20 years.

References

1. Boesch SM, Wenning GK, Ransmayr G, Poewe W. Dystonia in multiple system atrophy.
   J Neurol Neurosurg Psychiatry. 2002;72:300–3.
2. Askmark H, Edebol Eeg-Olofsson K, Johnsson A. Parkinsonism and neck extensor myopathy:
   a new syndrome or coincidental findings. Arch Neurol. 2001;58:232–7.

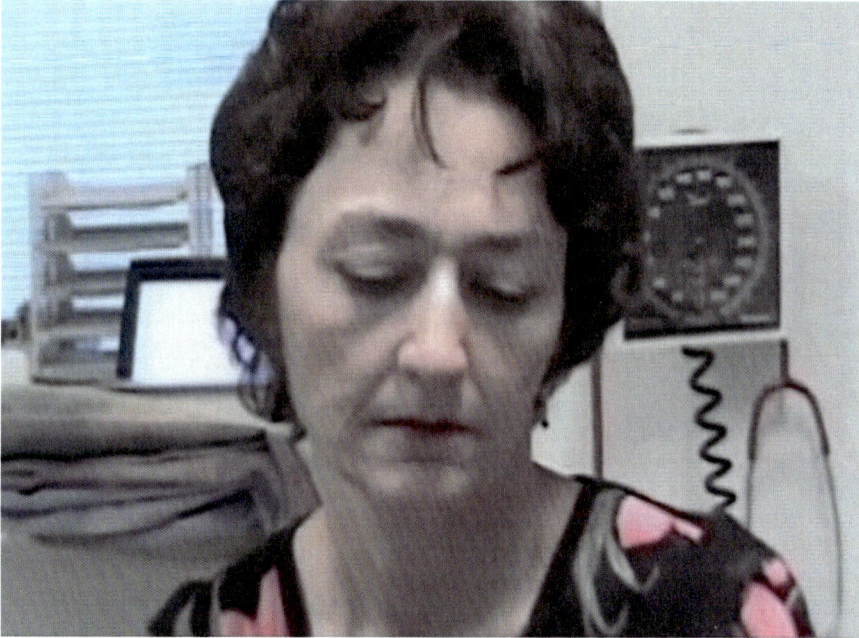

Video

The patient displays a mixed pattern of left laterocollis and torticollis. With eyes closed, she develops the slow appearance of anterocollis down and to the left side.

Chapter 42
Cervical Dystonia: Retrocollis

This chapter contains a video segment which can be found at the
URL: http://www.springerimages.com/Tarsy

Background

Retrocollis often occurs as a partial component of cervical dystonia and much less
commonly as an isolated manifestation (see Chap. 39). It may produce either a tonic
sustained retrocollic posture or may cause recurrent clonic vertical head jerks. When
part of a complex dystonia, it is more commonly associated with laterocollis than
other postural abnormalities. Isolated retrocollis is a common manifestation of tardive dystonia where it is commonly associated with extracervical dystonic manifestations and spasmodic head jerks.

Case

A 49-year-old woman developed the spontaneous appearance of mild left laterocollis followed within several months by much more severe retrocollis. There was no
history of treatment with antipsychotic medications or metoclopramide. She was
successfully treated with botulinum toxin type A for 8 years until she developed
antibody-mediated resistance. Treatment was switched to botulinum toxin type B
which has been followed to the present time by another 8 years of successful
treatment.

Reference

1. Molho ES, Feustel PJ, Factor SA. Clinical comparison of tardive and idiopathic cervical dystonia.
   Mov Disord. 1998;13:486–9.

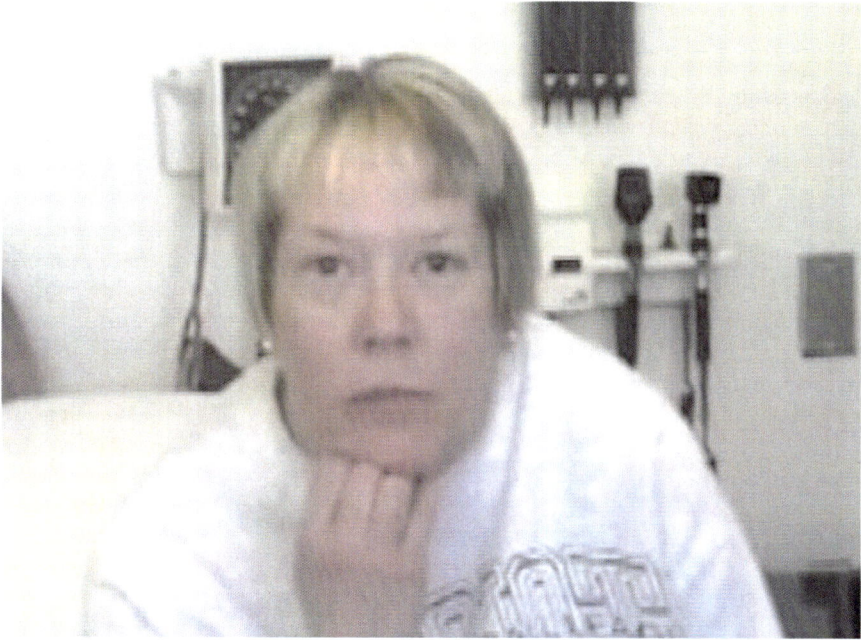

Video

The patient displays continuous tonic retrocollis together with a compensatory thoracic kyphosis. Vertical dystonic head jerks appear when she is asked to flex her neck. She displays an effective sensory trick with relief of retrocollis appearing just before and during placement of the fingers of her right hand beneath her chin (see Chap. 43).

Chapter 43
Cervical Dystonia: Sensory Tricks

This chapter contains a video segment which can be found at the
URL: http://www.springerimages.com/Tarsy

Background

Patients with different types of focal dystonia may experience temporary improvement of their dystonic symptoms with certain maneuvers, such as touching the chin,
cheek, or back of head in cervical dystonia; touching the eyelids in blepharospasm;
or touching the writing hand in writer's cramp. The "sensory trick" or "geste antag-
oniste" is a characteristic and unique feature and may serve as a diagnostic clue to
the diagnosis of focal dystonia. The most common form occurs in cervical dystonia
where placement of a finger on the chin may neutralize involuntary head movements. The tricks may be tactile or proprioceptive. Even imagining a particular
maneuver may diminish dystonic spasms. Although the presence of sensory tricks
in cervical dystonia occurs in up to 70% of cases, the mechanism of these tricks is
still unknown. Careful observation reveals that the "sensory tricks" are not simply a
counterpressure phenomenon. The diversity of effective maneuvers suggests that
higher sensorimotor integration processes are involved.

Case

A 46-year-old man, who had cervical dystonia for 2 years, experienced temporary
improvement of his dystonic symptoms by lightly touching his chin with one finger.
He adopted this maneuver into his daily routine when going to business meetings.
Examination showed dynamic retrocollic head movements with mild left laterocollis. However, his neck usually remained in neutral position when he placed his left
index finger on his chin.

References

1. Schramm A, Reiners K, Naumann M. Complex mechanisms of sensory tricks in cervical dystonia. Mov Disord. 2004;19:452–8.
2. Bhidayasiri R, Bronstein JM. Improvement of cervical dystonia: possible role of transcranial
magnetic stimulation simulating sensory tricks effects. Med Hypotheses. 2005;64:941–5.

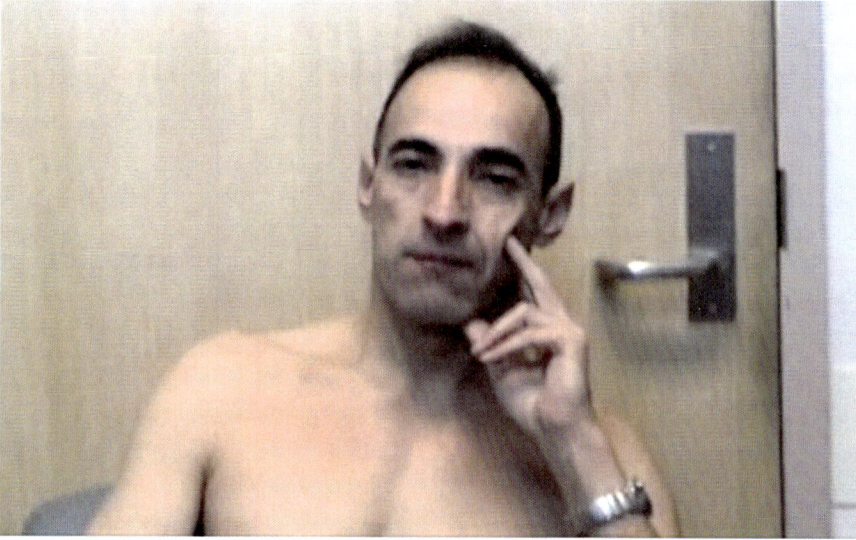

Video

The patient exhibits severe retrocollis with mild left laterocollis. He experiences significant pain when the dystonic jerks pull his neck backward. However, when he lightly places the fingers of his left hand on his chin, his neck remains in a nearly neutral position. Note that his neck begins to return to a neutral position even before he touches his chin, suggesting that the mechanism of the sensory trick is more than a simple counterpressure phenomenon.

Chapter 44
Secondary Cervical Dystonia Following Brainstem Hemorrhage

This chapter contains a video segment which can be found at the URL: http://www.springerimages.com/Tarsy

Background

Cervical dystonia (CD), also known as spasmodic torticollis, is the most common form of adult-onset focal dystonia. The vast majority of cases are idiopathic. Secondary cervical dystonia (SCD) is uncommon but can be associated with tardive dystonia, certain heredodegenerative neurologic disorders, vascular or neoplastic brain lesions, and trauma affecting the central or peripheral nervous system. Clues which favor secondary rather than idiopathic CD include fixed postures unaccompanied by involuntary head and neck movements and sensory tricks. Other focal neurologic findings may be present. Secondary cervical dystonia must be distinguished from nondystonic torticollis. Nondystonic torticollis refers to sustained muscle contractions often occurring in response to local neighborhood injuries or other abnormalities possibly as a reflex mechanism or reaction to another problem such as, for example, cervical disc herniation, atlantoaxial fractures or dislocations, cervical spine or spinal cord abnormalities, trochlear nerve palsy, or hemianopia. Abnormal head postures in neonates and children are almost never due to idiopathic CD and should be evaluated for nondystonic causes.

Structural brain lesions associated with cervical dystonia are most commonly localized to the brainstem and cerebellum. The remaining locations are in cervical spinal cord and basal ganglia. Adults with an acute or atypical presentation of CD such as severe pain, headache, nausea, vertigo, or other focal neurological signs should undergo imaging of the brain and cervical spine.

Case

A 51-year-old hypertensive man presented to the emergency room with the sudden onset of right-sided weakness and ataxia. Examination revealed right-sided weakness, severe bilateral appendicular ataxia which was worse on the right side, and right hemiparesthesia. Ocular examination revealed downbeat nystagmus in all directions of gaze. Brain CT scan showed a left pontine hemorrhage. One day later, he developed cervical dystonia with predominant right torticollis.

R. Bhidayasiri, D. Tarsy, *Movement Disorders: A Video Atlas*, Current Clinical Neurology, DOI 10.1007/978-1-60327-426-5_44, © Springer Science+Business Media New York 2012

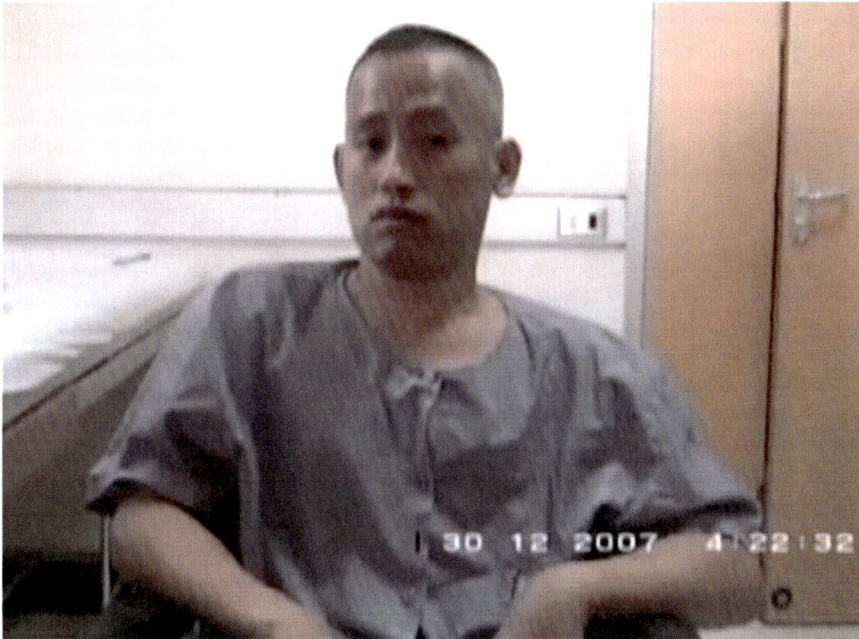

Video

One month after onset of symptoms, the patient displays right-sided torticollis with dynamic head jerks and bilateral upper extremity ataxia. There is hypertrophy of the left sternocleidomastoid muscle and mild right shoulder elevation.

References

1. LeDoux MS, Brady KA. Secondary cervical dystonia associated with structural lesions of the central nervous system. Mov Disord. 2002;18:60–9.
2. Suchowersky O, Calne DB. Nondystonic causes of torticollis. Adv Neurol. 1988;50:501–8.

Chapter 45
Secondary Hemidystonia Following Head Trauma

This chapter contains a video segment which can be found at the
URL: http://www.springerimages.com/Tarsy

Background

Head trauma is a well-recognized but infrequent cause of dystonia. Both hemidystonia and torticollis have been identified following head injury: Most patients (70%)
are men who have sustained severe head trauma with loss of consciousness. The
common presentation is that of acute hemiplegia followed by the delayed appearance of limb dystonia. The amount of delay may not correlate with severity of the
initial hemiparesis. Dystonia tends to progress as hemiparesis regresses. The onset
of dystonia may occur only days after trauma but sometimes is delayed for as long
as 6 years. Delayed onset is usually longer in children where it may occur as a con-
sequence of perinatal brain trauma. The young age and delayed onset of dystonia
suggest that the disorder represents an evolving process of neuronal plasticity and
may be due to neuronal reorganization.

Neuroimaging often identifies focal brain lesions in patients with posttraumatic
dystonia, particularly in those who present with hemidystonia. Pathoanatomical
correlations following head trauma are similar to those reported for secondary
hemidystonia due to other causes including lesions of the caudate, putamen, pallidum, and thalamus. Pontomesencephalic lesions have been reported in patients
with posttraumatic torticollis. Torticollis following brain injury differs from idiopathic cervical dystonia with typical features of secondary torticollis such as fixed
posture, limited cervical range of motion, absence of sensory tricks, persistence of
symptoms during sleep, predominant laterocollis, and a poor response to botulinum
toxin injections.

Case

A 21-year-old man who sustained a significant head injury in a motor vehicle accident 9 years previously was referred with increasingly severe jerking movements of
his right arm. The patient experienced right hemiparesis soon after the injury associated with significant cognitive dysfunction. Two weeks after the injury, tremor
appeared in his right arm which gradually worsened and coincided with stiffening
of his right arm and leg. Examination revealed a mild right hemiparesis, right upper
extremity tremor, and right hemidystonia mainly affecting the right arm. Brain MRI
showed small focal lesions in the left putamen together with diffuse evidence of old
cerebral trauma. No lesions were identified in brainstem, cerebellum, or thalamus.

R. Bhidayasiri, D. Tarsy, *Movement Disorders: A Video Atlas*, Current Clinical Neurology, 96
DOI 10.1007/978-1-60327-426-5_45, © Springer Science+Business Media New York 2012

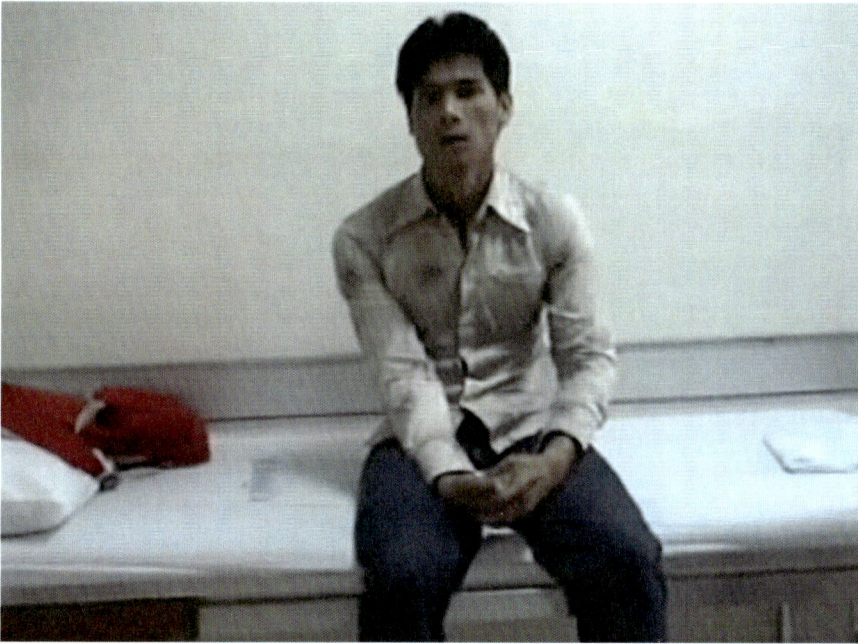

Video

An irregular and jerky large amplitude tremor is present in the right arm at rest which is worse with action. The patient also exhibits right hemidystonia which is most prominent in the right arm. The abnormal right arm posture is present at rest and becomes worse with action. Right facial pulling and mild right foot dystonia are also present. Mild right rotational torticollis is present together with hypertrophy of right sternocleidomastoid muscle. Gait is normal except for distal tremor in right arm and flexion dystonia at right wrist.

References

1. Krauss JK, Mohadjer M, Braus DF, et al. Dystonia following head trauma: a report of nine patients and review of the literature. Mov Disord. 1992;7:263–72.
2. Frei KP, Pathak M, Jenkins S, et al. Natural history of posttraumatic cervical dystonia. Mov Disord. 2004;19:1492–8.

Chapter 46
Essential Blepharospasm

This chapter contains a video segment which can be found at the
URL: http://www.springerimages.com/Tarsy

Background

Blepharospasm is a form of adult onset focal dystonia which is associated with
progressive involuntary spasms of the eyelid protractors including orbicularis oculi,
corrugator, and procerus muscles. The onset is usually in the fifth to seventh decade
of life with a female preponderance. Clinical presentations include increased blink
rate associated with photophobia and subjective feelings of ocular irritation, more
forceful exaggerated blinking, and delayed eyelid opening severe enough to cause
functional blindness known as "eyelid opening apraxia" (see Chap. 17). The spasms
may increase with bright light, reading, or watching television and may improve
while distracted with other physical tasks such as talking, humming, relaxation, or
gazing downward. Blepharospasm frequently coexists with other manifestations of
cranial dystonia, such as oromandibular dystonia, lower facial spasm, and anterocollis, and historically has been referred to as Meige syndrome (see Chap. 49).

In most patients, blepharospasm is unassociated with other neurologic disorders.
Some cases appear to be familial. An underlying cause is evident in approximately
14% of patients including Parkinson's disease, multiple system atrophy, progressive
supranuclear palsy, tardive dystonia, and occasional focal structural lesions in basal
ganglia, diencephalon, or upper brainstem. Botulinum toxin injections usually provide effective treatment for this condition.

Case

A 68-year-old woman presented to an outpatient eye clinic with complaints of photophobia, eye irritation, and spasmodic eye closure. The intensity and frequency of
spasms was increased by bright light, watching television, reading, and driving. The
spasms were sometimes so intense that driving was impossible. Examination
revealed increased blinking and frequent eyelid spasms. She found that applying a
light pressure on the temple or shutting one eye temporarily ameliorated the spasm.
There was no dystonia elsewhere.

R. Bhidayasiri, D. Tarsy, *Movement Disorders: A Video Atlas*, Current Clinical Neurology,
DOI 10.1007/978-1-60327-426-5_46, © Springer Science+Business Media New York 2012

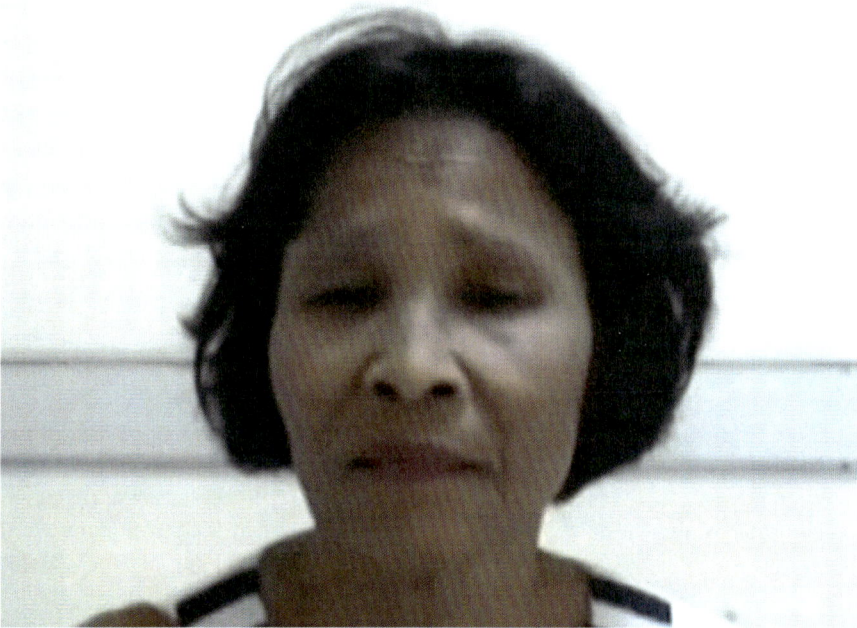

Video
The patient displays increased blink rate due to intermittent contractions of the orbicularis oculi muscles. There are also sustained contractions of the frontalis, nasalis, and corrugator muscles.

References

1. Grandas F, Elston J, Quinn N, et al. Blepharospasm: a review of 264 patients. J Neurol Neurosurg Psychiatry. 1988;51:767–72.
2. Defazio G, Abbruzzese G, Aniello MS, et al. Environmental risk factors and clinical phenotype in familial and sporadic primary blepharospasm. Neurology. 2011;77:631–7.

Chapter 47
Orofacial Dystonia and Dyskinesia

This chapter contains a video segment which can be found at the
URL: http://www.springerimages.com/Tarsy

Background

Orofacial dystonia and dyskinesia are associated with various combinations of spasmodic contractions of muscles of the jaw, lower face, lips, and tongue. Dystonic
movements are typically slower and more protracted while dyskinetic movements
are more frequent and rapid. Oromandibular dystonia (OMD) is perhaps the most
common of these and includes jaw opening, jaw closing, and jaw deviation dystonia. Facial dystonia usually involves the lower face and may produce puckering or
pursing movements of the mouth and lips, retraction or downward deviation of the
corners of the mouth, and puffing out of the cheeks. Embouchure dystonia is a task-
specific dystonia in which involuntary movements of the lips occur in wind instrument musicians only while playing their instruments. Other task-specific orofacial
dystonias may be activated by speaking or eating. Lingual dystonia produces involuntary movements of the tongue, the most disturbing of which is tongue protrusion.
In Meige syndrome, orofacial dystonia and dyskinesia are associated with blepharospasm and anterocollis is also often present (see Chap. 49). Differential diagnosis
includes tardive dystonia or dyskinesia in which similar perioral movements occur
following chronic exposure to antipsychotic drugs, random "mouthing" movements
which occur in elderly edentulous individuals with or without false teeth, and more
generalized disorders such as Lesch-Nyhan syndrome, neuroacanthocytosis, and
pantothenate kinase–associated degeneration in which oral dyskinesia is often
prominent. Painful forms of OMD are often mistaken for temporomandibular syndrome and bruxism. In jaw closing OMD, bruxism with clenching and grinding of
the teeth usually occurs when the patient is awake by contrast with nocturnal bruxism which occurs during sleep. Botulinum toxin injections into the masseters, ptery-
goid muscles, lingual muscles, or facial muscles are usually helpful. There are no
oral medications that appear to be effective.

Case

This 47-year-old man developed anteroflexion of his head and neck at age 37 followed shortly thereafter by increased eye blinking and pursing of his lips. At age 44,
anterocollis and blepharospasm spontaneously improved but he began experiencing
tongue protrusions, puckering postures of his lips, and jaw clenching, all of which
disturbed his speech. Examination showed slow, intermittent tongue protrusions,

R. Bhidayasiri, D. Tarsy, *Movement Disorders: A Video Atlas*, Current Clinical Neurology,   100
DOI 10.1007/978-1-60327-426-5_47, © Springer Science+Business Media New York 2012

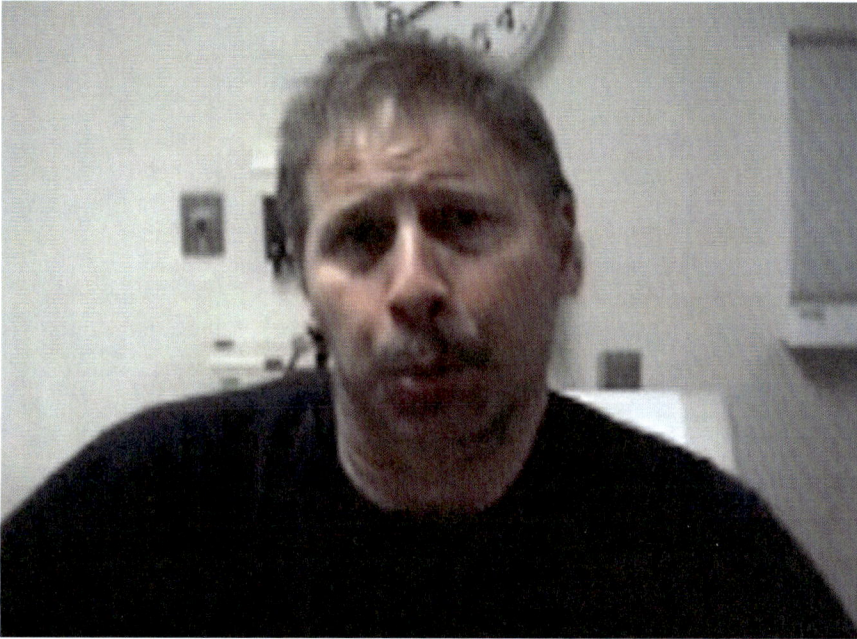

Video
The patient exhibits a pursing posture of his lips, small tongue protrusions, abnormal speech, mild right-side laterocollis with shoulder elevation, and increased frontalis creasing.

pursing of his lips, mild right laterocollis, and increased creasing in frontalis muscles. Botulinum toxin injections limited to genioglossus muscles reduced tongue protrusion.

References

1. Jankovic J, Ford J. Blepharospasm and orofacial-cervical dystonia: clinical and pharmacological findings in 100 patients. Ann Neurol. 1983;13:402–11.
2. Koller WC. Edentulous orodyskinesia. Ann Neurol. 1983;13:97–9.
3. Schneider SA, Aggarwal A, Bhatt M, et al. Severe tongue protrusion dystonia: clinical syndromes and possible treatment. Neurology. 2006;67:940–3.

Chapter 48
Orofacial Dystonia with Lower Facial and Platysma Dystonia

This chapter contains a video segment which can be found at the
URL: http://www.springerimages.com/Tarsy

Background

Lower facial dystonia produces abnormal movements and postures of the lower face
which are often associated with contractions of the platysma. Similar to other facial
dystonias which cause puckering or pursing of the lips, speech often activates the
movements thereby causing dysarthria. Lower facial dystonia is often accompanied
by anterocollis. Differential diagnosis is similar to other forms of orofacial dystonia
(see Chap. 47). Treatment is usually limited to injections of botulinum toxin into the
affected muscles. Care must be exercised with lower facial injections in order to
avoid lip closure weakness which may produce drooling.

Case

This 58-year-old man developed downward pulling at the corners of his mouth
bilaterally together with contractions of his platysma musculature at age 40. This
remained unchanged without other features of cranial dystonia. Botulinum toxin
into depressor labialis inferior and platysma has been effective in reducing distortion of the lower face and improving speech for a period of 18 years.

Reference

1. Jankovic J, Ford J. Blepharospasm and orofacial-cervical dystonia: clinical and pharmacological findings in 100 patients. Ann Neurol. 1983;13:402–11.

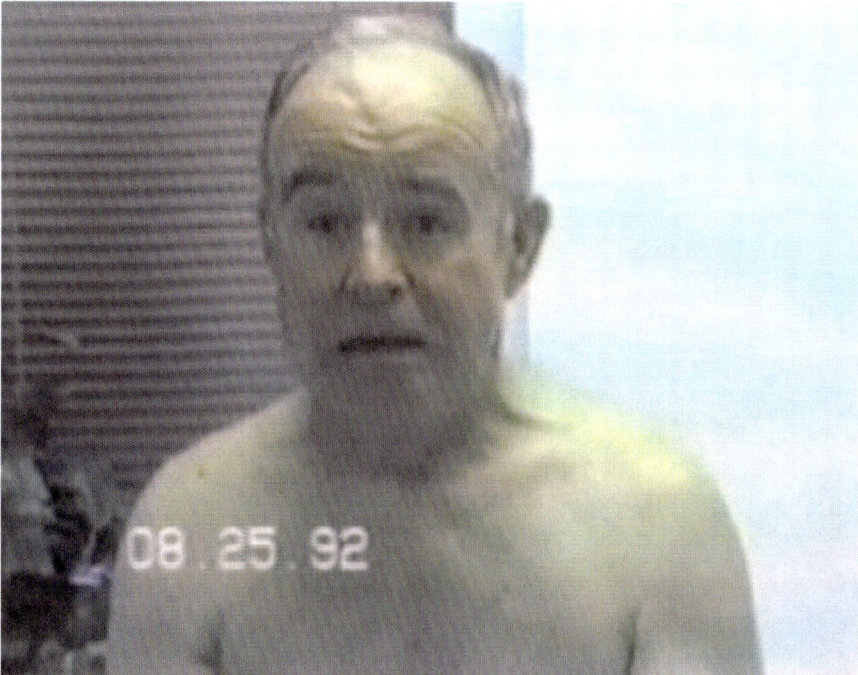

Video
While speaking, the patient displays downward contractions of the corners of his mouth and active contractions of the platysma.

Chapter 49
Meige's Syndrome

This chapter contains a video segment which can be found at the
URL: http://www.springerimages.com/Tarsy

Background

Meige syndrome refers to the combination of blepharospasm and orofacial dystonia. The term is mainly of historical interest having been described by Henry Meige
in 1910 but described by others prior to that including the Flemish painter Pieter
Bruegel the elder who portrayed affected individuals in several of his paintings.
Marsden C. David suggested that blepharospasm-oromandibular dystonia, like other
adult-onset focal dystonias, is a partial expression of primary dystonia and currently
is considered to be one of several forms of adult-onset focal dystonia. It is important
to recognize that many patients who display blepharospasm with orofacial dyskinesia are manifesting semi-voluntary movements of their lower face in a struggle to
keep their eyes open. In such cases, lower facial movements disappear after successful treatment of the blepharospasm with botulinum toxin. Lower facial and jaw
movements may include chewing, bruxism, jaw opening, lip and facial movements,
platysma contractions, and other forms of facial grimacing. In severe cases, chewing, swallowing, and speaking may be disturbed. Cervical dystonia, commonly in
the form of anterocollis, is often present. Women are affected more often than men
with mean age of onset of 50–60 years. Differential diagnosis includes secondary
cases, the most common of which is tardive dystonia due to chronic treatment with
antipsychotic medications. Blepharospasm should be distinguished from ptosis and
dry eye, while oromandibular dystonia should be distinguished from bruxism and
temporomandibular joint syndrome, both of which usually cause more pain than
occurs in jaw dystonia. Botulinum toxin into orbicularis oculi and jaw muscles is
the treatment of choice, while treatment with oral medications such as anticholin-
ergics and benzodiazepines is usually unhelpful.

Case

This 92-year-old woman first developed facial grimacing while in her 30s followed
by increased eyeblink frequency in her early 70s. Initial examination showed a combination of severe blepharospasm partially relieved by touching her upper lids with
her fingers, facial grimacing with retraction of the corners of her mouth, and
anteroflexion movements of her neck. The blepharospasm has been successfully
treated with eyelid botulinum toxin injections over a period of 20 years, while the
facial grimacing and anterocollis have persisted without change.

R. Bhidayasiri, D. Tarsy, *Movement Disorders: A Video Atlas*, Current Clinical Neurology,
DOI 10.1007/978-1-60327-426-5_49, © Springer Science+Business Media New York 2012

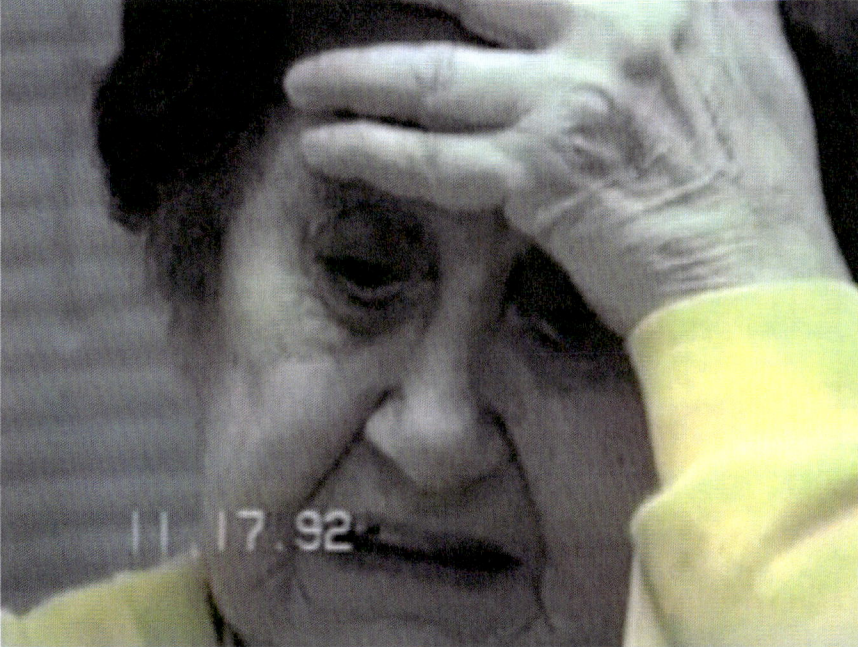

Video
The patient exhibits involuntary blepharospasm, lower facial grimacing, and anterocollis.

References

1. Meige H. Les convulsions de la face: une forme Clinique de convulsions facials, bilaterale et mediane. Rev Neurol (Paris). 1910;21:437–43.
2. Marsden C. David Blepharospasm-oromandibular dystonia syndrome (Bruegel's syndrome): a variant of adult-onset torsion dystonia? J Neurol Neurosurg Psychiatry. 1976;59:1204–9.
3. Tolosa ES, Klawans HL. Meige's disease: a clinical form of facial convulsion, bilateral and medial. Arch Neurol. 1979;36:635–7.

Chapter 50
Tongue Protrusion Dystonia

This chapter contains a video segment which can be found at the
URL: http://www.springerimages.com/Tarsy

Background

Orobuccal-lingual dystonia is characterized by involuntary movements of muscles
of the lower face, mouth, and tongue. It is one of the primary adult-onset focal dystonias but is also often present in patients with heredodegenerative or secondary
forms of dystonias. Neuroacanthocytosis, pantothenate kinase–associated neurodegeneration, Lesch-Nyhan syndrome, tardive dystonia, and postanoxic dystonia are
all commonly associated with oral dystonia. Severe forms of tongue dystonia may
be life threatening and management can be very challenging. Oral medications for
dystonia are nearly always ineffective. Botulinum toxin injections into the genioglossus muscles which protrude the tongue may be helpful and usually does not
cause swallowing difficulty. Globus pallidum deep brain stimulation may be considered in very disabled patients.

Case

A 38-year-old woman was referred because of intermittent severe episodes of tongue
protrusion. She had previously been treated with high dosages of anticholinergic
drugs, clonazepam, and baclofen without success. Examination showed severe
intermittent tongue protrusion associated with jaw-opening dystonia. Blepharospasm
was also present. Dystonia was present in the upper extremities causing difficulty
with handwriting and eating. She denied any history of neuroleptic exposure.
Extensive investigations including neuroimaging, blood smear for acanthocytes,
ceruloplasmin, copper, and iron studies were unrevealing. She was believed to have
a spontaneous lingual dystonia.

References

1. Schneider SA, Aggrawal A, Bhatt M, et al. Severe tongue protrusion dystonia clinical syndromes and possible treatment. Neurology. 2006;67:940–3.
2. Charles PD, Davis TL, Shannon KM, et al. Tongue protrusion dystonia: treatment with botulinum toxin. South Med J. 1997;90:522–5.

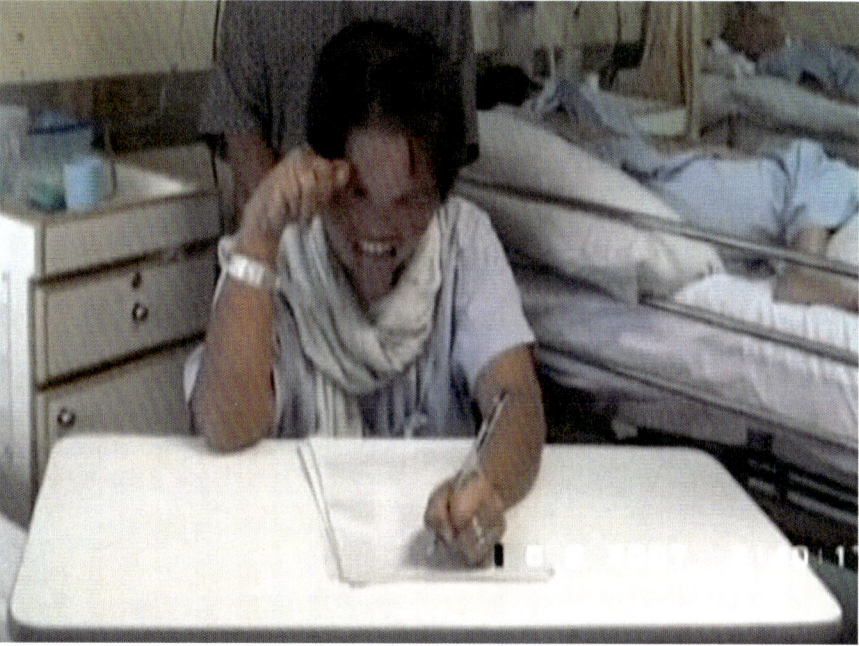

Video
The patient exhibits severe tongue protrusion dystonia associated with jaw-opening dystonia and blepharospasm. Dystonia is present in upper extremities bilaterally and is exacerbated while writing.

Chapter 51
Spasmodic (Laryngeal) Dysphonia

This chapter contains a video segment which can be found at the
URL: http://www.springerimages.com/Tarsy

Background

Spasmodic dysphonia (SD) is an adult-onset focal dystonia characterized by abnormal vocal cord contractions activated by speech. There are three forms of spasmodic dysphonia. The commonest form, making up about 90% of cases, is adductor dysphonia in which spasmodic adduction of the vocal cords causes interruptions in phonation called voice breaks. Because of the resultant closed glottis speech is highly strained, effortful, high-pitched, and reduced in volume. Whispering is often normal. The second most common type is abductor dysphonia in which patients have a breathy voice with aphonic interruptions occurring in the middle of a word. These typically occur when phonating a vowel right after a voiceless consonant such as a p, f, s, t, or h. The third type is the least common and is due to a mixture of these. Compensatory tricks to overcome the voice abnormality are common and may include whispering and humming. Adductor laryngeal breathing dystonia is an uncommon variant of laryngeal dystonia characterized by inspiratory stridor which occurs only while awake and is unaccompanied by a voice abnormality. Differential diagnosis is very limited and includes primary disturbances of the larynx and voice tremor. Many patients with SD are incorrectly diagnosed as having a psychological basis for their symptoms. The diagnosis is usually made by listening to the voice, sometimes supplemented by fiberoptic laryngoscopy which shows excessive speech-activated vocal cord adduction in adductor dysphonia and excessive speech-activated abduction in abductor dysphonia. The treatment of choice is unilateral or bilateral botulinum toxin injections into the thyroarytenoid muscles for adductor dysphonia and cricothyroid or posterior cricoarytenoid injections for abductor dysphonia. There are no effective oral medications for this condition and voice therapy is nearly always ineffective.

Case

This 63-year-old operating room nurse began with voice difficulty at age 45 following an uncomplicated sinus infection. Voice pattern has included a combination of voice strain and voice breaks, has remained unchanged for 18 years, and is unassociated with any other focal dystonia. She has been treated with botulinum injections into thyroarytenoid muscles every 4–6 months with excellent responses.

R. Bhidayasiri, D. Tarsy, *Movement Disorders: A Video Atlas*, Current Clinical Neurology, 108
DOI 10.1007/978-1-60327-426-5_51, © Springer Science+Business Media New York 2012

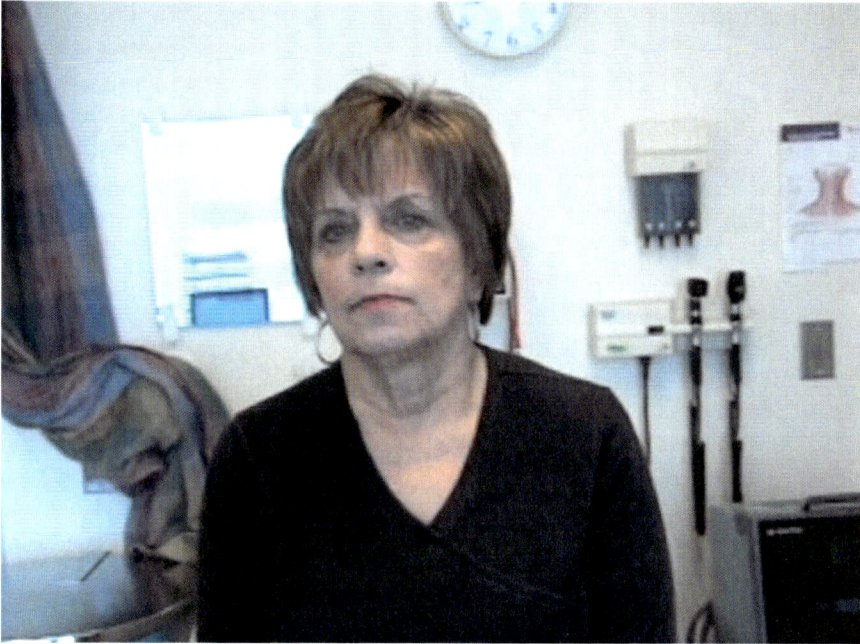

Video
Patient exhibits a staccato style voice pattern. She can whisper and sing relatively normally.

References

1. Ludlow CL, Naunton RF, Sedory SE, Schulz GM, Hallett M. Effects of botulinum toxin injections on speech in adductor spasmodic dysphonia. Neurology. 1988;38:1220–5.
2. Whurr R, Lorch M, Fontana H, et al. The use of botulinum toxin in the treatment of adductor spasmodic dysphonia. J Neurol Neurosurg Psychiatry. 1993;56:526–30.
3. Grillone GA, Blitzer A, Brin M, Annino DJ, Saint-Hilaire MH. Treatment of adductor laryngeal breathing dystonia with botulinum toxin type A. Laryngoscope. 1994;104:30–2.
4. Truong DD, Bhidayasiri R. Botulinum toxin therapy of laryngeal muscle hyperactivity syndromes: comparing different botulinum toxin preparations. Eur J Neurol. 2006;13 Suppl 1:36–41.

Chapter 52
Writer's Cramp

This chapter contains a video segment which can be found at the
URL: http://www.springerimages.com/Tarsy

Background

Writer's cramp (WC) is a form of task-specific focal dystonia which causes excessive contractions of the muscles of the forearm and hand activated by writing. Other motor tasks of the hand may become affected over time, at which point it is referred to as dystonic writer's cramp. WC is a subtype of other occupational cramp disorders, the best known of which is musician's cramp occurring in pianists or string players. WC was originally described in individuals whose occupation demanded unusually large amounts of writing but may also occur in the absence of excessive writing. Forearm pain and a variety of abnormal postures of the hand and fingers are observed within moments of beginning to write such as excessive flexion of the fingers or thumb, excessive wrist flexion, or hyperextension of one or more digits. An excessively strong grip on the pen is usually apparent, and in some cases the elbow may elevate from the writing surface. Writing is often slow and effortful indicative of an associated disorder of motor control. When asked to write with the opposite hand, the dominant hand may exhibit mirror movements which display the dystonic postures of the affected hand. Writing is usually normal while using more proximal muscles to write on a blackboard or easel. It sometimes occurs as a presenting or relatively isolated sign in *DYT1* dystonia or dopa-responsive dystonia. Differential diagnosis includes "overuse" syndromes in which arm and hand pain may occur with excessive writing but is unaccompanied by dystonic posture. Genetic factors probably play a significant role since a family history of other forms of focal dystonia is present in up to 20% of cases. Disturbed sensory discrimination and an enlarged cortical representation of the affected hand and digits have been reported, although it is unclear if this is etiologically important or simply an accompaniment of excessive hand activity. Treatment of choice is botulinum toxin injections into the hyperactive muscles, but this is not always effective due to unwanted weakness of adjacent muscles or inability to significantly improve disturbed motor control. Use of special writing implements is sometimes helpful.

Case

A college administrator developed involuntary extensor posturing of his index finger while writing at age 26. His job did not demand a great deal of writing. About 10 years later, similar difficulty appeared while playing the guitar. One of his brothers has hand

R. Bhidayasiri, D. Tarsy, *Movement Disorders: A Video Atlas*, Current Clinical Neurology,
DOI 10.1007/978-1-60327-426-5_52, © Springer Science+Business Media New York 2012

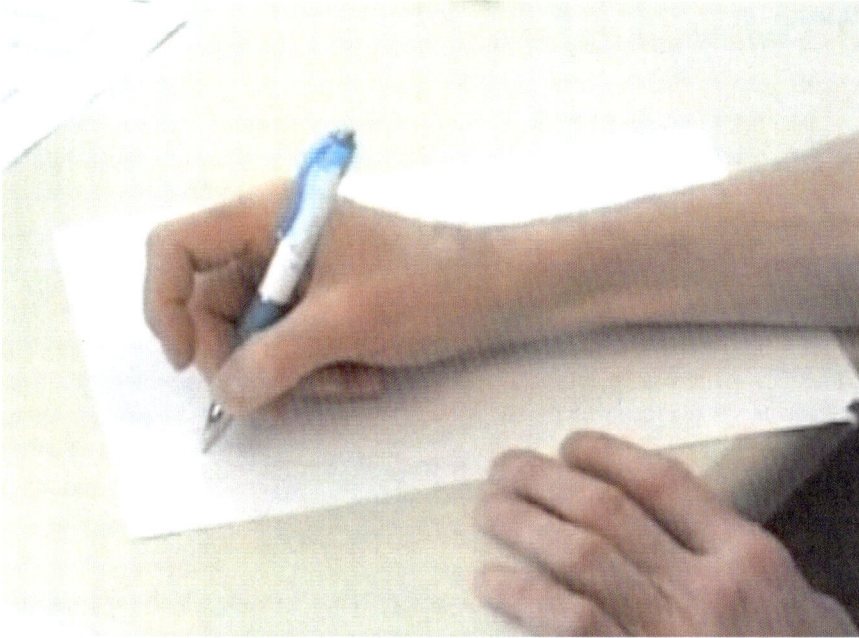

Video
The patient exhibits involuntary extension at the metacarpophalangeal joint of the index finger while writing.

tremor and several family members have been observed to hold a glass with their index finger extended. He has had successful treatment with injections of relatively small doses of botulinum toxin into extensor indicis proprius over a period of 16 years.

References

1. Sheehy MP, Marsden CD. Writer's cramp: a focal dystonia. Brain. 1982;105:461–80.
2. Cohen LG, Hallett M. Hand cramps: clinical features and electromyographic patterns in a focal dystonia. Neurology. 1988;38:1005–12.
3. Bara-Jimenez W, Shelton P, Sanger TD, et al. Sensory discrimination capabilities in patients with focal hand dystonia. Ann Neurol. 2000;47:377–80.

Chapter 53
Writer's Cramp with Mirror Movements

This chapter contains a video segment which can be found at the
URL: http://www.springerimages.com/Tarsy

Background

Motor overflow refers to unintentional muscle contractions which accompany but
are anatomically separate from primary involuntary dystonic movements. In the
case of writer's cramp, mirror movements are a form of overflow in which abnormal
movements occur in the unoccupied affected hand while writing with the opposite
unaffected hand. This phenomenon suggests the presence of more widespread
abnormalities of motor control in patients with focal dystonia, possibly due to a loss
of normal inhibitory mechanisms. When looked for in individuals with writer's
cramp, the appearance of mirror dystonia in the affected resting hand is common
when writing with the opposite unaffected hand. From a practical viewpoint, it is
particularly helpful to be able to elicit and more clearly display dystonic movements
and postures when the symptomatic hand is not engaged in writing.

Case

An 18-year-old student with a 3-year history of writer's cramp was referred for
botulinum toxin injections. She had become unable to write in class. In order to
compensate for her writing difficulty, she had started to type on a notebook computer. Examination of her right hand while writing revealed flexion dystonia of the
wrist and fingers. Similar but less severe mirror dystonia was observed in the right
hand while writing with her unaffected left hand.

References

1. Sitburana O, Wu LJC, Sheffield JK, et al. Motor overflow and mirror dystonia. Parkinsonism
   Relat Disord. 2009;15:758–61.
2. Espay AJ, Li J-Y, Johnston L, et al. Mirror movements in parkinsonism: evaluation of a new
   clinical sign. J Neurol Neurosurg Psychiatry. 2005;76:1355–9.
3. Merello M, Carpintiero S, Cammarota A, et al. Bilateral mirror writing movements (mirror
   dystonia) in a patient with writer's cramp: functional correlates. Mov Disord. 2006;21:683–9.

R. Bhidayasiri, D. Tarsy, *Movement Disorders: A Video Atlas*, Current Clinical Neurology,   112
DOI 10.1007/978-1-60327-426-5_53, © Springer Science+Business Media New York 2012

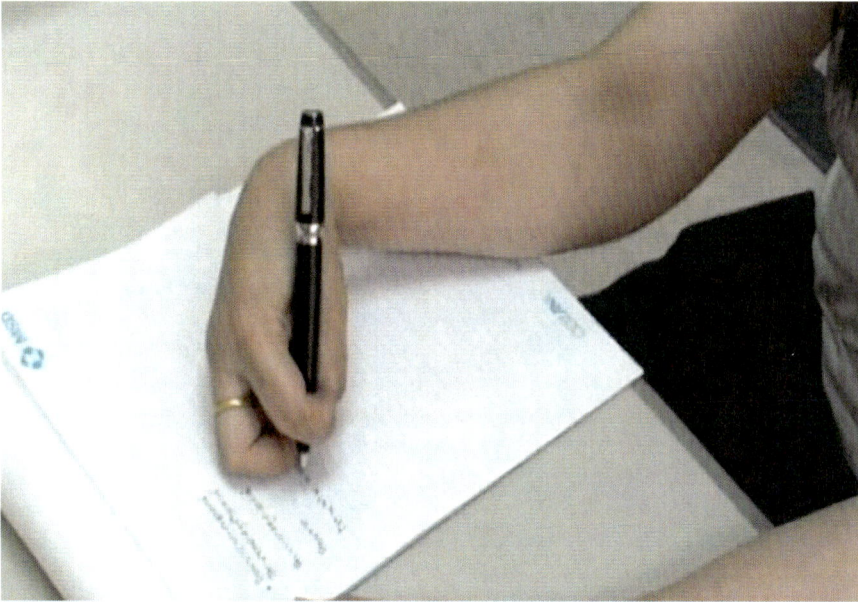

Video

Clip 1: the patient attempts to write with her dominant right hand. She exhibits severe flexion dystonia of the right wrist and fingers with ipsilateral overflow to the elbow and shoulder regions. Writing is intermittently interrupted due to severe cramps in her right hand. *Clip 2*: the patient begins to write with her unaffected left hand and within seconds develops mirror dystonia in the right hand manifested by flexion of the right wrist and fingers.

Chapter 54
Musician's Dystonia in a Guitarist

This chapter contains a video segment which can be found at the
URL: http://www.springerimages.com/Tarsy

Background

Focal dystonia in musicians, known as musician's cramp or musician's dystonia, is
a task-specific movement disorder which causes a loss of muscular coordination and
voluntary motor control of extensively trained, highly skilled movements while
playing a musical instrument (see Chap. 55). Musician's dystonia may be classified
according to the musical tasks which are affected. Embouchure dystonia affects the
coordination of lips, tongue, and facial and cervical muscles in brass and wind players. Pianist's or violinist's cramp affects control of finger, hand, or arm movements.
It is estimated that approximately 1% of professional musicians are affected by this
disorder. A higher risk has been observed in musicians who play instruments requiring extremely fine motor skills. Typically, musician's dystonia occurs without pain,
although muscle aching may occur after prolonged spasms. Focal dystonia appears
more commonly in the more intensely used hand. Initial loss of muscular coordination is followed by co-contraction of agonist and antagonist muscle groups. Etiology
is poorly understood, but the following predisposing factors have been proposed:
male gender, positive family history of focal dystonia, increased high intensity prac-
ticing, traumatic injury to the affected body part, musical and social constraints
typical of the performance situation in classical music, and underlying anxiety and
perfectionism. Botulinum toxin injections are often considered but responses in
professional musicians are usually disappointing due to demands for a perfect outcome and concerns for unwanted weakness. Prolonged rest is typically unhelpful
unless there is an accompanying overuse syndrome. In many cases, the disorder has
terminated the career of affected musicians.

Case

A 25-year-old professional guitarist was referred for a suspected nerve injury to his
left hand. The patient's main complaint was aching of the fingers of his left hand
during prolonged playing unaccompanied by pain or numbness. Due to financial
pressures, he was working 7 days weekly in a local bar playing for up to 6 h daily.
Examination at rest was unremarkable. When playing his guitar, flexion dystonia
was observed mainly in the left index finger but may also have involved the fourth
and fifth fingers. There were no signs of dystonia elsewhere.

R. Bhidayasiri, D. Tarsy, *Movement Disorders: A Video Atlas*, Current Clinical Neurology, 114
DOI 10.1007/978-1-60327-426-5_54, © Springer Science+Business Media New York 2012

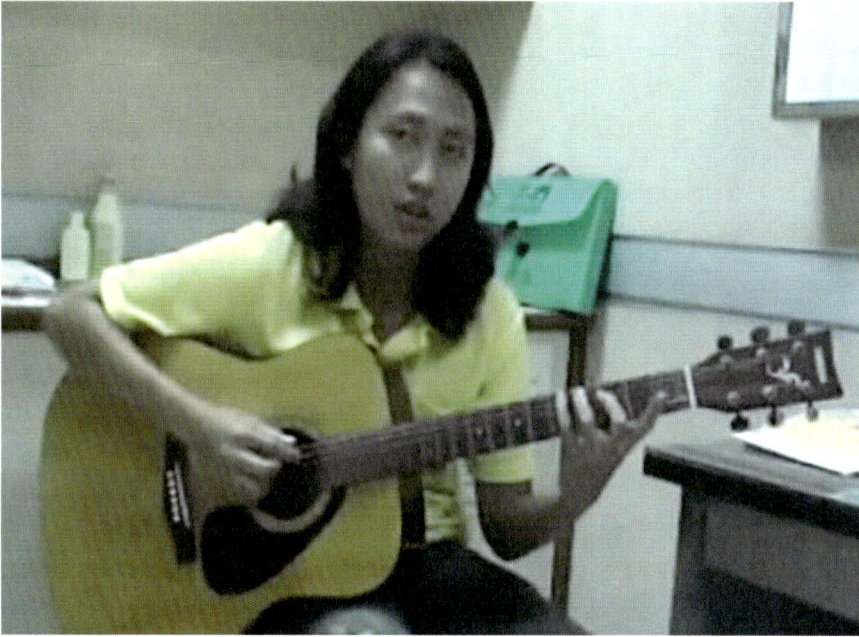

Video
Clip 1: the patient exhibits extension dystonia predominantly in his left index finger and less so in the left fourth and fifth fingers. *Clip 2*: another example of musician's dystonia in a pianist with flexion dystonia affecting several digits of the right hand.

References

1. Altenmuller E, Jabusch H-C. Focal dystonia in musicians: phenomenology, pathophysiology and triggering factors. Eur J Neurol. 2010;17 Suppl 3:31–6.
2. Jankovic J, Ashoori A. Movement disorders in musicians. Mov Disord. 2008;23:1957–65.

Chapter 55
Musician's Dystonia in a Violinist

This chapter contains a video segment which can be found at the
URL: http://www.springerimages.com/Tarsy

Background

Musician's dystonia is a form of task-specific dystonia in which the ability to play a
musical instrument is impaired by focal dystonia precipitated exclusively by playing the instrument (see Chap. 54). Violinist's or pianist's dystonia most commonly
affects the fourth and fifth fingers of one hand but may also affect the wrist and arm.
Embouchure dystonia affects coordination of the lips, tongue, and facial muscles in
brass and wind players. In the case of violinist's dystonia, impaired coordination is
noticed first followed by abnormal posturing of the fingers or hand. It often appears
during a period of high-intensity practice which often drives the musician to further
increase practice time. Botulinum toxin injections into appropriate muscles are usually recommended and may be helpful but responses are often disappointing because
of the high demand for perfection typically sought by professional musicians.
Prolonged rest and splinting are typically unhelpful unless there is also a component
of overuse syndrome.

Case

This 33-year-old right-handed professional violinist was referred following a 1-year
history of difficulty playing the violin. This first began with rapid passages demand-
ing quicker finger movements. Six months previously, she increased practice to 8 h
daily preparing for a series of auditions. She then switched to a smaller violin and
at that time noticed that the fourth and fifth fingers of her left hand were curling
involuntarily while playing. The effect on her playing was subtle and not noticed by
her colleagues. These symptoms did not occur while using her left hand for other
manual activities. Her family, which includes three other professional musicians,
has no history of focal dystonia. On examination, while playing the violin, she displayed repeated flexion posturing of the fourth and fifth fingers of her left hand. This
cleared as soon as she stopped playing and was not present at rest or while writing,
drawing, or carrying out other motor tasks with that hand. Her examination was
otherwise normal. To date, she has deferred botulinum toxin and is trying to modify
her playing style to accommodate the dystonia.

R. Bhidayasiri, D. Tarsy, *Movement Disorders: A Video Atlas*, Current Clinical Neurology,
DOI 10.1007/978-1-60327-426-5_55, © Springer Science+Business Media New York 2012

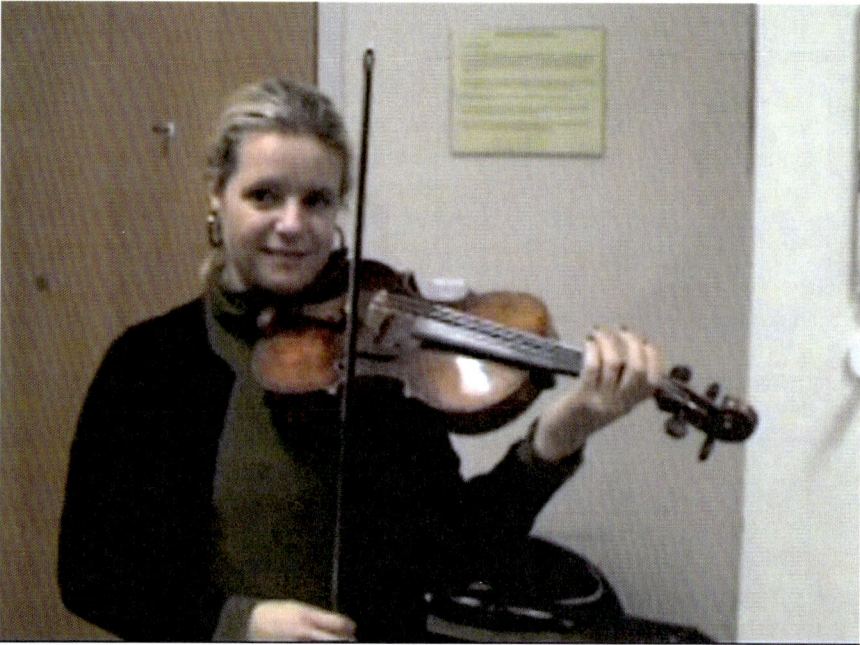

Video
Flexion posturing of fourth and fifth fingers appears very shortly after beginning to play the violin. It stops when she is not playing the violin.

References

1. Altenmuller E, Jabusch H-C. Focal dystonia in musicians: phenomenology, pathophysiology and triggering factors. Eur J Neurol. 2010;17:31–6.
2. Jankovic J, Ashoori A. Movement disorders in musicians. Mov Disord. 2008;23:1957–65.

Chapter 56
Rower's Dystonia

This chapter contains a video segment which can be found at the
URL: http://www.springerimages.com/Tarsy

Background

Task-specific action dystonia, also known as occupational cramp, is a focal dystonia
which is absent at rest and occurs only during the performance of repetitive, highly
skilled movements. Currently, the most common task-specific dystonias are writer's
cramp and musician's dystonia. The condition has also been described among rec-
reational athletes including pistol-shooters, dart throwers, long-distance runners,
table tennis players, and golfers. These are uncommon disorders which often go
undiagnosed for long periods of time. Here we describe a case of task-specific action
dystonia in a competitive rower. This appears to be a task-specific action dystonia
because of its exclusive occurrence during performance of a skilled motor task, its
occurrence after a prolonged period of intensive training, and the absence of any
contributory neurologic or orthopedic abnormalities. Though the cause of task-
specific action dystonia is unknown, abnormal cortical mechanisms of inhibition
and plasticity may play a role in its pathogenesis (see Chap. 52). No genetic abnormality has been associated with these dystonias, but there is an increased incidence
of other types of focal dystonia in the families of affected individuals.

Case

Following 3 years of intense training, a 22-year old competitive rower experienced
right-sided incoordination which compromised his performance. He described a
"hitch" in his right arm and difficulty properly planting his right foot while pulling
back on his oar. No involuntary movements or abnormal postures occurred during
other routine motor activities. There was no family history of dystonia or any other
movement disorder. Physical therapy and chiropractic treatment were unhelpful. He
was referred for a movement disorders consultation. Neurological examination was
normal with no signs of dystonia at rest. While observed using a portable rowing
machine, he displayed immediate and persistent hyperabduction of his right arm
while pulling back on his oar as well as inability to fully plant the toes of his right
foot during each stroke. Serum ceruloplasmin, brain and cervical spine MRI, and
electromyography were normal. Levodopa 25/100 mg three times daily was unhelpful. He declined botulinum toxin because of his concern that it would cause arm and
shoulder weakness.

R. Bhidayasiri, D. Tarsy, *Movement Disorders: A Video Atlas*, Current Clinical Neurology, 118
DOI 10.1007/978-1-60327-426-5_56, © Springer Science+Business Media New York 2012

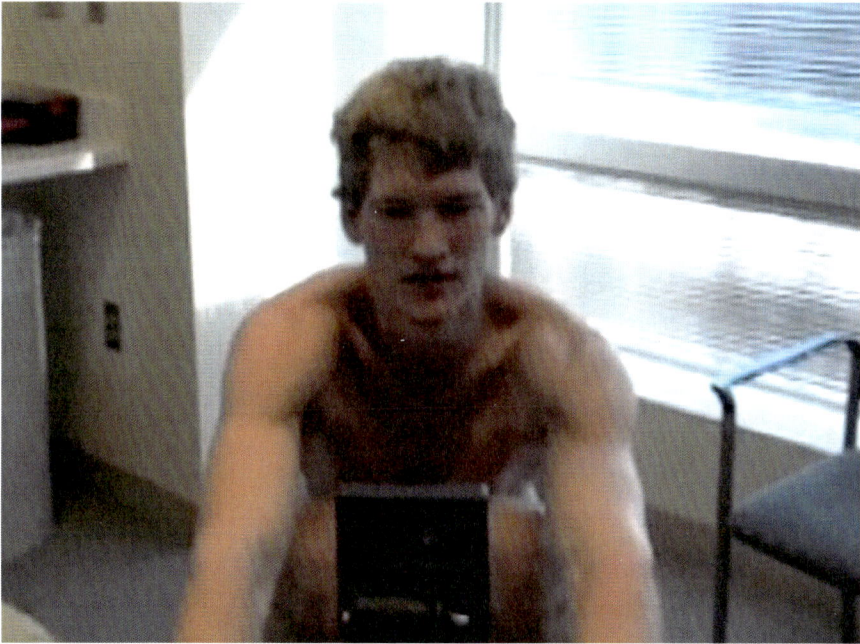

Video
Hyperabduction of the right upper arm and failure to fully plant the toes of the right foot are evident during the backstroke.

References

1. Torres-Russotto D, Perlmutter JS. Task-specific dystonias: a review. Ann NY Acad Sci. 2008;1142:179–99.
2. Le Floch A, Vidhailet M, Flamand-Rouviere C, et al. Table tennis dystonia. Mov Disord. 2010;25:394–7.

Chapter 57
Neurodegeneration with Brain Iron Accumulation

This chapter contains a video segment which can be found at the
URL: http://www.springerimages.com/Tarsy

Background

Neurodegeneration with brain iron accumulation (NBIA) encompasses a group of
progressive extrapyramidal disorders which are characterized by the accumulation of
brain iron. The term NBIA is now widely used in the medical literature and is
sufficiently broad to encompass the spectrum of disorders previously called
Hallervorden-Spatz disease as well as other disorders causing elevated levels of brain
iron such as neuroaxonal dystrophy, neuroferritinopathy, and aceruloplasminemia.

The major form of NBIA is pantothenate kinase–associated neurodegeneration
(PKAN), formerly known as Hallervorden-Spatz disease, which is caused by mutations in the *PANK2* gene. PKAN accounts for approximately 50% of cases of NBIA.
Aceruloplasminemia, caused by mutations in the CP gene, and neuroferritinopathy,
caused by mutations in the *FTL* gene, make up a small proportion of other cases of
NBIA. Recent studies suggest that both infantile neuroaxonal dystrophy and atypical neuroaxonal dystrophy are caused by mutations in the *PLA2G6* gene and, in
about half of the cases, also result in high brain iron accumulation.

Classic PKAN is characterized by early onset, often before age 6, and rapid
progression. Affected children often appear clumsy before the onset of frank
symptoms such as abnormal gait due to dystonia. Primary clinical features include
dystonia, dysarthria, rigidity, and spasticity. Pigmentary retinal degeneration is
common. Attention deficit hyperactivity disorder is commonly diagnosed prior to
recognition of PKAN. Atypical cases occur at a later age of onset (13–14 years)
and are associated with slower disease progression. In PKAN, a central region of
hyperintensity in the globus pallidus with surrounding hypointensity on T2W
images known as the "eye of the tiger" is virtually pathognomonic for this disease
(Fig. 57.1). A correlation has been established between this MRI finding and the
presence of a *PANK2* mutation.

Case

A 25-year-old man presented with a 7-year history of slowly progressive gait
difficulty characterized by stiffness of his legs and trunk. He walked with short
shuffling steps. Examination disclosed axial and cervical dystonia together with
spasticity and brisk reflexes in both lower extremities. Brain MRI showed the "eye
of the tiger" sign (Fig. 57.1).

R. Bhidayasiri, D. Tarsy, *Movement Disorders: A Video Atlas*, Current Clinical Neurology,
DOI 10.1007/978-1-60327-426-5_57, © Springer Science+Business Media New York 2012

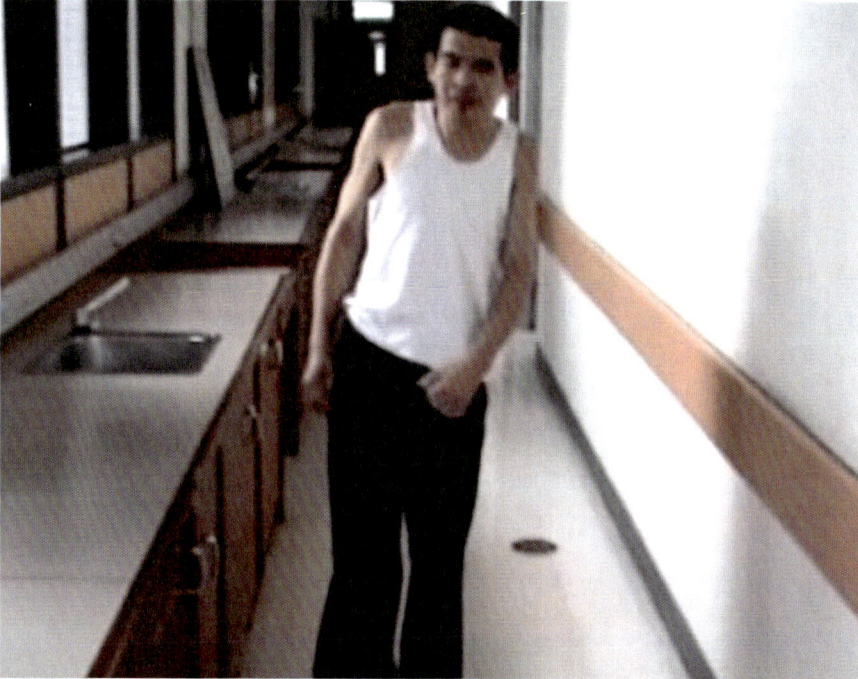

Video

The patient has generalized dystonia which predominantly affects the trunk and cervical regions. Episodes of dystonic spasm are evident when he sits upright and walks. Gait is characterized by short stride length and shuffling together with elbow flexion and shoulder abduction.

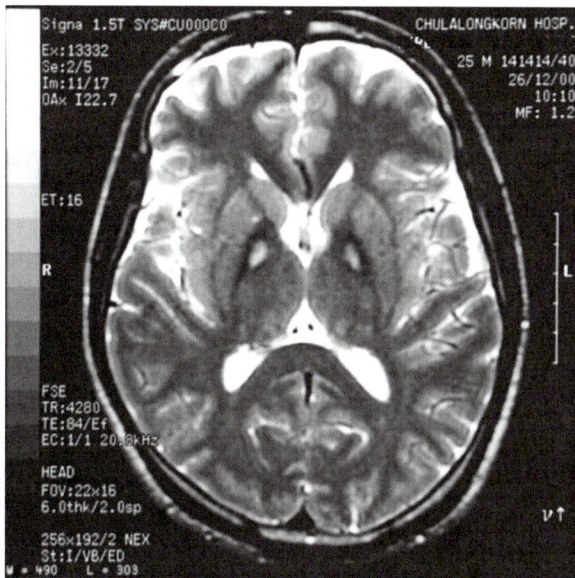

Fig. 57.1 T2-weighted brain MRI showed a central hyperintensity lesion, surrounded by hypointensity region in the globus pallidus, known as "eye of the tiger" sign.

References

1. Gregory A, Polster BJ, Hayflick SJ. Clinical and genetic delineation of neurodegeneration with brain iron accumulation. J Med Genet. 2009;46:73–80.
2. Hayflick SJ, Westaway SK, Levinson B, et al. Genetic, clinical, and radiographic delineation of Hallervorden-Spatz syndrome. N Eng J Med. 2003;348:33–40.

Chapter 58
Spinocerebellar Ataxia-Type 2 with Dystonia

This chapter contains a video segment which can be found at the
URL: http://www.springerimages.com/Tarsy

Background

Spinocerebellar ataxia type 2 (SCA2) is an autosomal dominant cerebellar ataxia
that commonly presents with ataxia, slow saccadic eye movements, dysarthria, and
peripheral neuropathy. Extremely slow saccades are common but not pathognomonic. The expanded CAG repeat is SCA2 which encodes polyQ in the abnormal
gene product, ataxin-2 (see Chap. 98). Normal alleles are between 15 and 32 repeats
in length while expanded alleles are 53–77 repeats in length. Together with SCA6,
SCA2 is the form most likely to occur sporadically without a positive family history
in prior generations. This is believed to be due to further expansion of a modestly
enlarged repeat during transmission from one generation to the next.

In some individuals with SCA2, extrapyramidal movement disorders such as parkinsonism and dystonia have been prominent. These are regarded as manifesting the
parkinsonism predominant SCA2 phenotype. Parkinsonism in SCA2 may be indistinguishable from idiopathic Parkinson's disease (PD) including improvement with
levodopa therapy and occurrence of levodopa-related motor complications. This
finding is consistent with postmortem studies which have shown prominent basal
ganglia abnormalities in addition to severe atrophy of the cerebellum and brainstem.
Recently, cervical dystonia has been reported to be one of the more common and
even presenting features of SCA2 and may precede ataxia and gait disturbance.

Case

A 53-year-old woman initially presented with blepharospasm followed later by
severe retrocollis which had been present for the past year. The dystonia had progressed to produce hyperextension of the back resulting in gait difficulty. There was
no family history of similarly affected members. Examination showed marked retrocollis, left laterocollis, and axial dystonia manifest by hyperextension of the trunk
which caused a tendency to fall backward. The SCA2 gene contained 36 repeats.

R. Bhidayasiri, D. Tarsy, *Movement Disorders: A Video Atlas*, Current Clinical Neurology,
DOI 10.1007/978-1-60327-426-5_58, © Springer Science+Business Media New York 2012

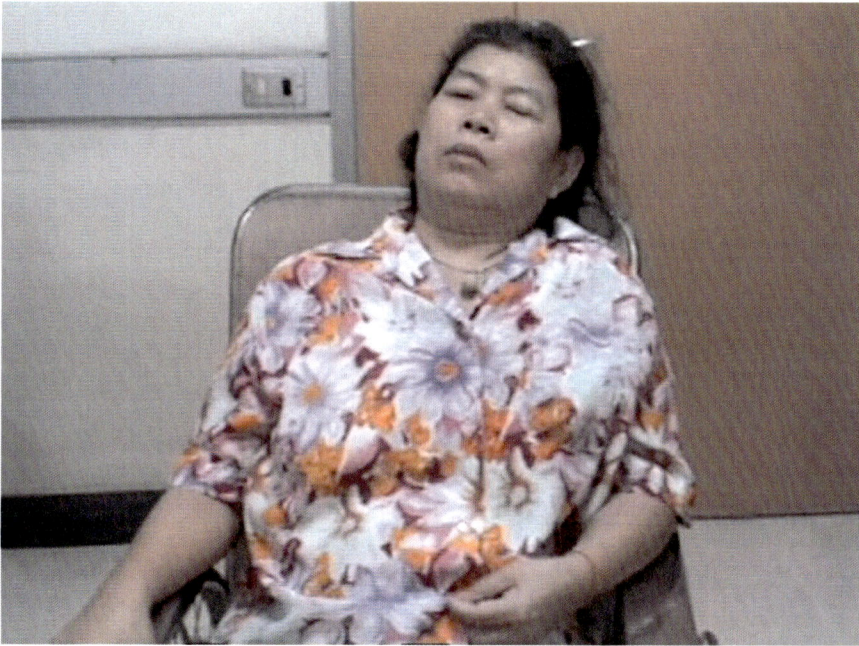

Video
The patient exhibits severe retrocollis, left laterocollis, and elevation of the left shoulder with muscle jerks. Axial dystonia is prominent while walking manifest by opisthotonic posturing which contributes to a tendency to fall backward. (Video contribution from Dr. Priya Jagota, Chulalongkorn Center of Excellence on Parkinson's Disease and Related Disorders, Thailand).

References

1. Klockgether T. The clinical diagnosis of autosomal dominant cerebellar ataxias. Cerebellum. 2008;7:101–5.
2. Furtado S, Payami H, Lockhart PJ, et al. Profiles of families with parkinsonism-predominant spinocerebellar ataxia type 2 (SCA2). Mov Disord. 2004;19:622–9.
3. Boesch SM, Muller J, Wenning GK, et al. Cervical dystonia in spinocerebellar ataxia type 2: clinical and polymyographic findings. J Neurol Neurosurg Psychiatry. 2007;78:520–2.

Chapter 59
Tardive Dystonia

This chapter contains a video segment which can be found at the
URL: http://www.springerimages.com/Tarsy

Background

Tardive dystonia (TD) refers to involuntary dystonic movements and postures
which, like tardive dyskinesia (see Chap. 77), are due to the chronic use of dopamine receptor blocking agents (DRBAs) such as antipsychotic drugs and metoclopramide. Young adults appear to be particularly susceptible to this disorder. Although
choreiform movements may occur, the principal feature is dystonia which must be
present for more than a month and occur either during ongoing treatment with a
DRBA or within 3 months of its discontinuation. Dystonic movements in TD differ
from classical tardive dyskinesia in several ways: (1) They commonly involve axial
muscles of the neck and trunk; (2) they tend to be more action specific, occurring
intermittently with certain actions or postures and without exhibiting the more regular periodicity of classical tardive dyskinesia; (3) dystonic movements can sometimes be partially suppressed by simple sensory tricks; (4) unlike tardive dyskinesia,
TD occurs more often among men than women.

Without a reliable drug history, TD may be indistinguishable from idiopathic
torsion dystonia. However TD has a special predilection for cervical and truncal
muscles and more often produces retrocollis or opisthotonus. Internal rotation of the
arms, hyperextension of the elbows, and flexion of the wrists are particularly common postures. The legs are less commonly involved.

Case

A 57-year-old man with long history of neuroleptic treatment was referred for botulinum toxin injections for neck spasms. He reported a gradual stiffening of the neck
and trunk muscles over the previous 3 years. Examination disclosed retrocollis and
truncal dystonia, which tended to pull him backward while sitting or walking.

References

1. Bhidayasiri R, Boonyawairoj S. Spectrum of tardive syndromes: Recognition and management.
   Postgrad Med J. 2011;87:132–41.
2. Kang UJ, Burke RE, Fahn S. Natural history and treatment of tardive dystonia. Mov Disord.
   1986;1:193–208.
3. Tarsy D, Bralower M. Tardive dyskinesia in young adults. Am J Psychiatry. 1977;134:1032–4.

R. Bhidayasiri, D. Tarsy, *Movement Disorders: A Video Atlas*, Current Clinical Neurology,   126
DOI 10.1007/978-1-60327-426-5_59, © Springer Science+Business Media New York 2012

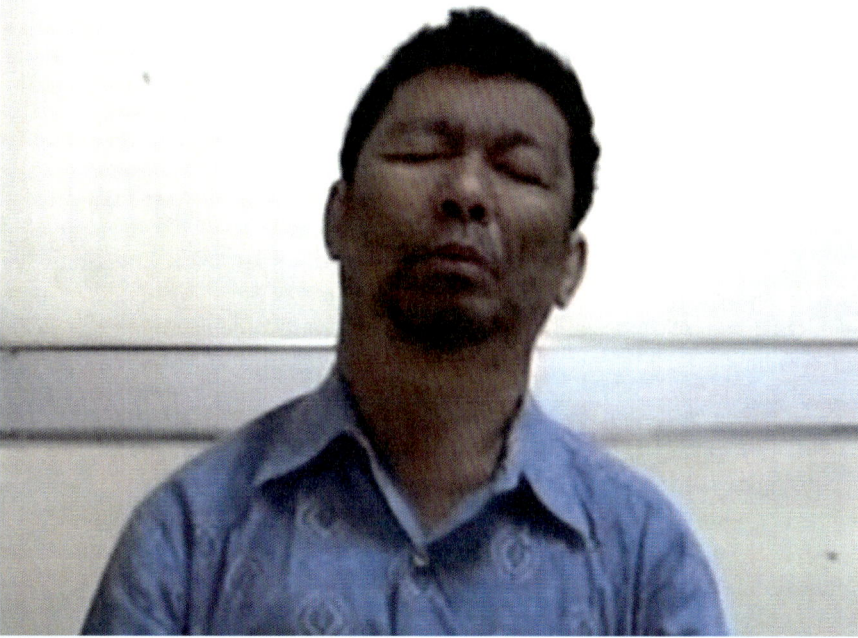

Video
The patient displays retrocollis and left laterocollis. Orobuccal dystonia and dyskinesia are evident together with blepharospasm. Mild truncal dystonia and scoliosis are also present. His legs are minimally affected.

Chapter 60
Tardive Dystonia Treated with Deep Brain Stimulation

This chapter contains a video segment which can be found at the
URL: http://www.springerimages.com/Tarsy

Background

Tardive dystonia (TD) refers to involuntary dystonic movements and postures
which, like tardive dyskinesia (see Chap. 59), are due to the chronic use of dopamine receptor blocking agents (DRBAs) such as antipsychotic drugs and metoclopramide. Young adults appear to be particularly susceptible to this disorder. Although
choreiform movements may occur, the principal feature of TD is dystonia which
must be present for more than a month and occur either during ongoing treatment
with DRBAs or within 3 months of its discontinuation. Dystonic movements in TD
differ from classical tardive dyskinesia in several ways: (1) They typically involve
axial muscles of the neck and trunk; (2) they tend to be more action specific, occurring intermittently with certain actions or postures and without exhibiting the more
regular periodicity of classical tardive dyskinesia; (3) dystonic movements can
sometimes be partially suppressed by simple sensory tricks; (4) unlike tardive dyskinesia, TD occurs more often among men than women. TD has a special predilection for cervical and truncal muscles and often produces retrocollis or opisthotonus.
Internal rotation of the arms, hyperextension of the elbows, and flexion of the wrists
are other common dystonic postures. The legs are less commonly involved.
Treatment options include withdrawal of DRBAs, anticholinergic drugs, botulinum
toxin injections, tetrabenazine, and globus pallidus deep brain stimulation (DBS).
Notably, the clinical response to DBS in patients with TD has been much more rapid
in onset than in patients with other forms of dystonia.

Case

This 50-year-old man presented with a 10-year history of TD occurring on a background of chronic bipolar disorder since age 25 which had been treated with antipsychotic drugs since onset. TD had always consisted of retrocollis, which was his
most disabling symptom, together with axial dystonia and abnormal postures of his
upper extremities. Examination showed spasmodic retrocollis with synchronous
jerks of his upper trunk together with retraction of his jaw, facial grimacing, jaw
clenching, blepharospasm, and internal rotational dystonic movements in both
upper extremities. He was taking thiothixene at the time which was discontinued
with mild worsening of his dystonia. Botulinum injections into posterior cervical

muscles produced only mild relief of retrocollis. He underwent bilateral globus pallidus DBS, and within 2 days of initial programming, there was marked improvement in all aspects of his dystonia except for mild oral and upper extremity dyskinesia. Burke-Fahn-Marsden dystonia score improved from 35 to 3.

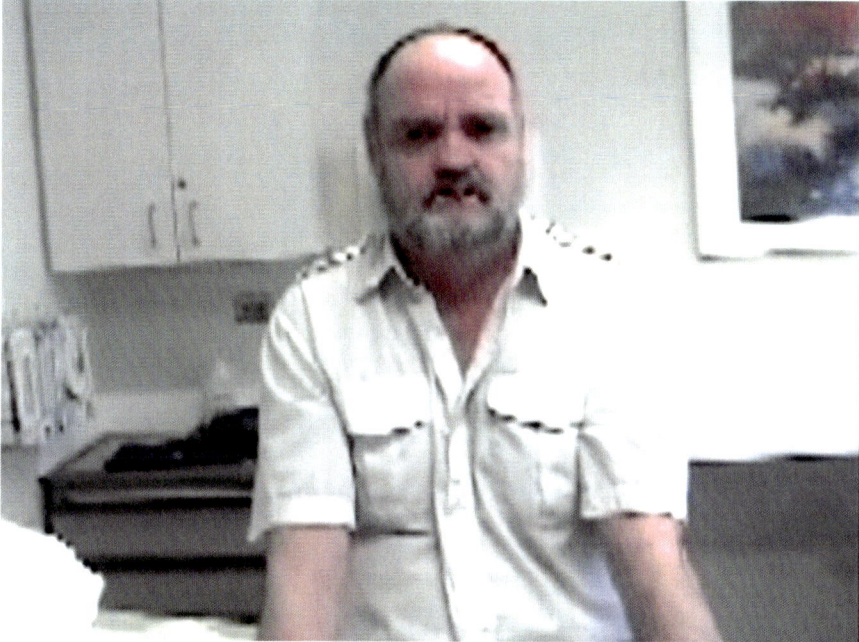

Video

Clip 1: prior to DBS, the patient exhibits spasmodic retrocollis with synchronous jerks of the upper trunk. There is retraction of his jaw, facial grimacing, jaw clenching, and blepharospasm. Internal rotational dystonic movements are present distally in both upper extremities. *Clip 2*: four weeks after DBS, neck and trunk are now quiet, and there is no facial grimacing or upper extremity dystonia. There is mild retrocollis with eyes closed and arms extended.

References

1. Kang UJ, Burke RE, Fahn S. Natural history and treatment of tardive dystonia. Mov Disord. 1986;1:193–208.
2. Tarsy D, Bralower M. Tardive dyskinesia in young adults. Am J Psychiatry. 1977;134:1032–4.
3. Sako W, Goto S, Shimazu H, et al. Bilateral deep brain stimulation of the globus pallidus internus in tardive dystonia. Mov Disord. 2008;23:1929–31.
4. Gruber D, Trottenberg T, Kivi A, et al. Long-term effects of pallidal deep brain stimulation in tardive dystonia. Neurology. 2009;73:53–8.

Chapter 61
Wilson's Disease with Dystonia

This chapter contains a video segment which can be found at the
URL: http://www.springerimages.com/Tarsy

Background

Wilson's disease is an autosomal recessive disorder caused by mutations in the
ATP7B gene, resulting in abnormal copper metabolism with toxic accumulation of
copper. Clinical manifestations vary considerably. It has been said that "there is
only one thing which all these patients have in common, apart from the Kayser-
Fleischer ring, and that is that they are all different." Since treatment can cure
Wilson's disease, early disease recognition is of paramount importance as it can
lead to the initiation of appropriate and effective therapy. Wilson's disease should be
considered in adolescents and adults younger than age 40 with the following features: (1) elevated liver enzymes found incidentally or in the context of an acute
episode of hepatitis; (2) dysphagia or dysarthria not explained by another neurological disorder; (3) any type of unexplained movement disorder; (4) psychiatric symptoms with liver disease; (5) adolescents with mood disorders and minor elevation of
liver transaminase; (6) Coombs-negative hemolytic anemia; and (7) unexplained
liver cirrhosis or hepatic failure. Clinical manifestations of neurologic Wilson's disease include variable combinations of dysarthria together with abnormal movements such as dystonia, tremor, parkinsonism, and/or choreoathetosis.

Dystonia is commonly present in patients with Wilson's disease with a prevalence of 11–65%. A frequent dystonic manifestation is the dystonic facial expression known as risus sardonicus which creates a fixed and exaggerated smile.
Jaw-opening dystonia and focal dystonia of the vocal cords, muscles of articulation,
and swallowing frequently cause dysphonia, dysarthria, and dysphagia. Dystonia
typically begins unilaterally but may progress to become more generalized. The
presence of dystonia correlates with MRI signal abnormalities in the putamen.

Case

A 28-year-old man with no significant previous medical history was brought to the
psychiatric emergency room because of aggressive behavior and confusion. History
obtained from his girlfriend suggested that his erratic behavior began at age 19 and
was characterized by multiple emotional outbursts, depression, and auditory halluci-
nations. He was diagnosed with bipolar disorder 5 years earlier. During the past year,
he began walking more slowly and speaking with a softer voice. He complained of
stiffness in his extremities. His psychiatrist's initial impression was drug-induced

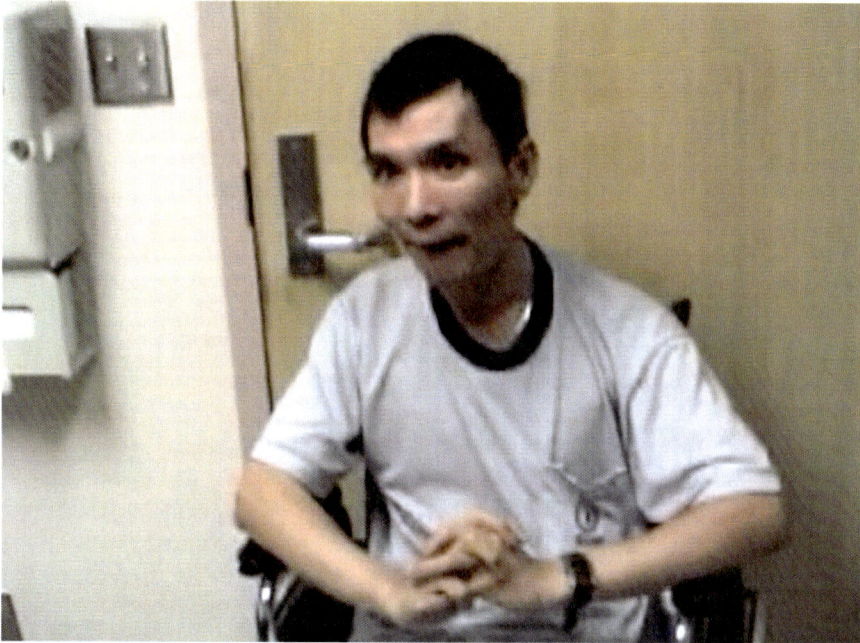

Video
The patient exhibits a risus sardonicus. There is generalized dystonia including predominant jaw-opening dystonia. His speech is dysarthric. There is dystonic posturing of the hands and toes. Both legs are dystonic and spastic with brisk reflexes.

parkinsonism. Examination revealed soft and slow speech associated with drooling. A risus sardonicus was evident. His jaw remained open most of the time. Generalized dystonia with spasticity made him unable to stand or walk.

References

1. Walshe JM. Wilson's disease: yesterday, today, and tomorrow. Mov Disord. 1988;3:10–29.
2. Bull PC, Thomas GR, Rommens JM, et al. The Wilson disease gene is a putative copper transporting P-type ATPase similar to the Menkes gene. Nat Genet. 1993;5:327–37.

Chapter 62
Rapid-Onset Dystonia Parkinsonism

This chapter contains a video segment which can be found at the
URL: http://www.springerimages.com/Tarsy

Background

Rapid-onset dystonia parkinsonism (RDP) is a rare autosomal dominant disorder
that usually affects adolescents and young adults but occasionally young children.
It begins abruptly and evolves very rapidly over days to weeks. A typical onset is
with orofacial dystonia, severe dysarthria, dysphagia, and muscle cramps in upper
extremities associated with variable degrees of bradykinesia, rigidity, and postural
instability. Cranial and upper limb muscles are more affected than the lower limbs.
Bulbar involvement is prominent manifest by an open mouth, drooling, and near
inability to speak or swallow. Initial deficits usually stabilize over the first few weeks
but may then persist unchanged or show mild improvement. Possible triggers which
have been reported include vigorous exercise, fever, heat exposure, and psychological stress. In some cases, residual focal dystonia has been followed years later by
reappearance of sudden bulbar and other motor symptoms. RDP is due to a mis-
sense mutation in *ATP1A3*, the gene on chromosome 19q13 encoding the α3 sub-
unit of the Na/K-ATPase pump. Rarely new mutations in *ATP1A3* have been reported
in individuals with no family history of RDP. There are no readily available diagnostic tests for RDP. The diagnostic test is identification of a mutation in the *ATP1A3*
gene. Treatments with levodopa, dopamine agonists, anticholinergic drugs, and pallidotomy have usually been ineffective. Pathological examination of one case
revealed no brain abnormalities.

Case

A 29-year-old woman had developed a step wise appearance of flexion dystonia of
the left hand, arm, and foot over a period of 3 years. Examination showed fixed
dystonic rigidity of the left fingers, hand, and elbow and a more fluid focal dystonia
of the left leg and foot which produced mild gait abnormality. Treatment with tri-
hexiphenidyl produced mild benefit, but when discontinued 1.5 years later, she
developed sudden dysarthria, difficulty moving her facial muscles, dysphagia, and
increased gait disturbance in the context of a urinary tract infection. She evolved
over the next week to being unable to speak with more severe dysphagia.
Laryngoscopic examination showed adduction weakness and irregular involuntary
movements of the vocal cords. Her left-sided dystonia was unchanged.

R. Bhidayasiri, D. Tarsy, *Movement Disorders: A Video Atlas*, Current Clinical Neurology,
DOI 10.1007/978-1-60327-426-5_62, © Springer Science+Business Media New York 2012

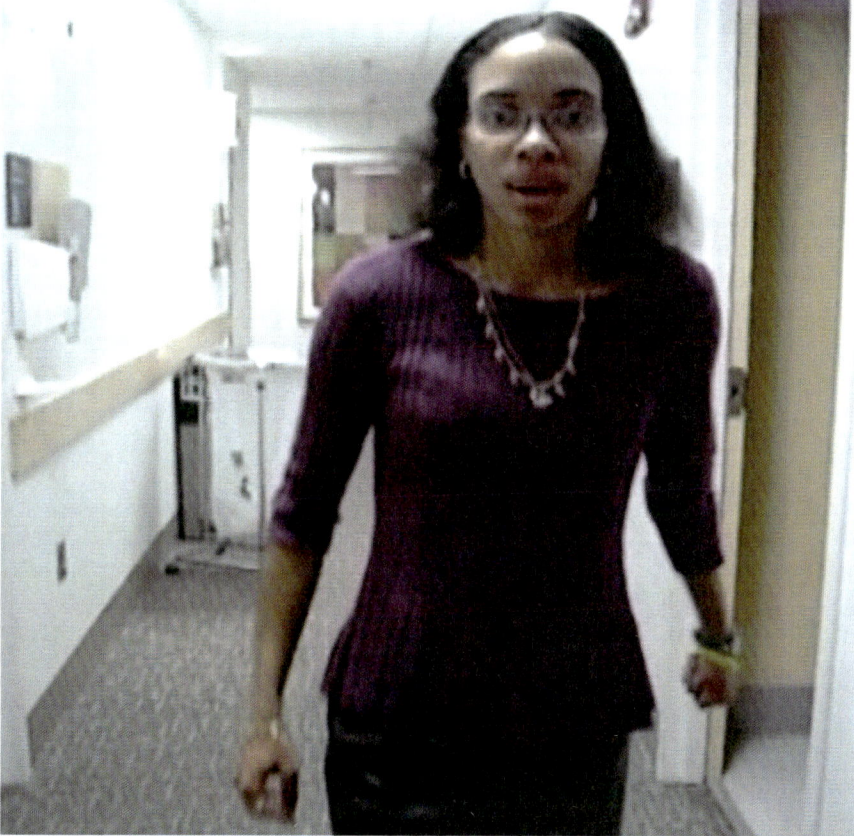

Video
Clip 1: the patient has a stiff gait with reduced arm swing. Facial expression is markedly reduced. *Clip 2*: the same patient exhibits fixed flexion dystonia of left hand. (Video contribution from Dr. Nutan Sharma, Massachusetts General Hospital, Boston.)

References

1. Brashear A, DeLeon D, Bressman SB, et al. Rapid-onset dystonia-parkinsonism in a second family. Neurology. 1997;48:1066–9.
2. Brashear A, Dobyns WB, de CArvalho Aguiar P, et al. The phenotypic spectrum of rapid-onset dystonia-parkinsonism (RDP) and mutations in the *ATP1A* gene. Brain. 2007;130:828–35.
3. Tarsy D, Sweadner KJ, Song PC. Case 17–2010: a 29-year-old woman with flexion of the left hand and foot and difficulty speaking. N Engl J Med. 2010;362:2213–9.

Chapter 63
Anterocollis in Parkinsonism

This chapter contains a video segment which can be found at the
URL: http://www.springerimages.com/Tarsy

Background

Disproportionate anterocollis in parkinsonism refers to forward flexion of the head
and neck which is greater than expected relative to the flexed posture of the trunk and
limbs. Anterocollis has been described in idiopathic Parkinson's disease (PD) and
multiple system atrophy (MSA) but rarely in progressive supranuclear palsy or diffuse Lewy body disease. Indeed, the presence of this sign in a patient with parkinsonism is regarded as a "red flag" which should raise the possibility of MSA.
Interestingly, anterocollis has not been reported in young-onset PD despite its long
disease duration. The etiology of anterocollis is poorly understood but neck extensor
myopathy, unbalanced rigidity of anterior and posterior neck muscles, "off-period
dystonia" in levodopa-responsive patients with PD, and dopamine agonists have all
been suggested. In cases due to extensor myopathy of neck muscles, this condition is
called "dropped head syndrome." In cases which are due to dystonia, the sternocleidomastoid, levator, and/or longus colli muscles are overactive. Electromyography
may be useful in identifying dystonic spasm in these muscles or in identifying myo-
pathic changes in paraspinal neck extensor muscles. Anterocollis affects the patient's
ability to speak, swallow, see, and communicate and also causes drooling and neck
pain, further impairing quality of life.

Case

The family of a 75-year-old man with an 8-year history of PD observed that his neck
had become more stooped, resulting in difficulty speaking and swallowing. In addition, he drooled because of "difficulty in keeping saliva in my mouth." Examination
revealed severe neck flexion while flexed posture elsewhere was mild. Neck flexion
was fixed making examination of neck muscles difficult but no apparent neck extensor weakness was present. However, relative hypertrophy of cervical paraspinal and
bilateral sternocleidomastoid muscles was present. Unfortunately, electromyography was not performed in this patient.

R. Bhidayasiri, D. Tarsy, *Movement Disorders: A Video Atlas*, Current Clinical Neurology, 134
DOI 10.1007/978-1-60327-426-5_63, © Springer Science+Business Media New York 2012

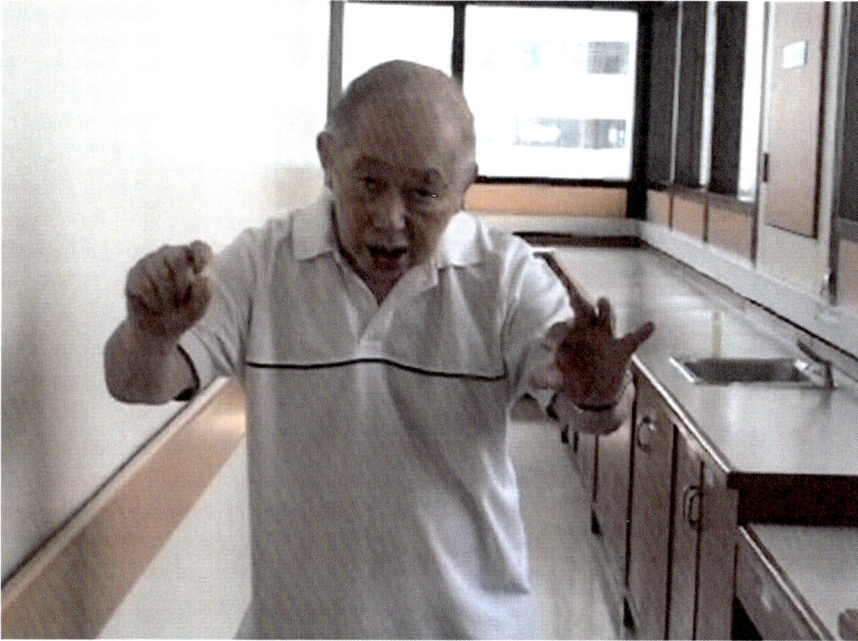

Video

Clip 1: examination shows marked facial masking and neck flexion. Right hand tremor is present while standing and walking. *Clip 2*: examination of another patient, a woman with anterocollis, illustrates severe neck flexion and anterior shift of the head. While supine, neck flexion resolves and she is able to lie flat.

References

1. van de Warrenberg BPC, Cordivari C, Ryan AM, et al. The phenomenon of disproportionate antecollis in Parkinson's disease and multiple system atrophy. Mov Disord. 2007;22:2325–31.
2. Quinn N. Disproportionate antecollis in multiple system atrophy. Lancet. 1989;1(8642):844.

Chapter 64
Sandifer's Syndrome

This chapter contains a video segment which can be found at the
URL: http://www.springerimages.com/Tarsy

Background

Sandifer's syndrome refers to a disorder which causes gastro-esophageal reflux and
abnormal posturing. Although the precise mechanism is unclear, it is hypothesized
that the positioning of the head and upper extremities adopted by the affected child
provides relief from the abdominal discomfort caused by acid reflux. Thought to be
a rare disorder, Sandifer's syndrome typically occurs during infancy and early childhood. The abnormal movements are usually manifest as nodding head movements,
rotations and extension postures of the head and neck, gurgling sounds, writhing
movements of the limbs, and severe hypotonia. Intermittent stiff tonic postures and
episodic crying and discomfort may suggest seizures, although evidence to support
this possibility is lacking. Symptoms beginning shortly after feeding should suggest
this diagnosis. Investigations often reveal marked hiatal hernia (although not essential for this disorder), erosive esophagitis, malnutrition, and chronic anemia. The
causal relation between gastro-esophageal reflex and abnormal posturing is supported by the resolution of the manifestations after successful treatment of reflux
disease. Half of the cases require fundoplication surgery for definitive therapy.

Case

A 6-year-old boy was referred for the treatment of dystonia. Extensive investigations since age 2 were unrevealing. However, there were frequent episodes of
abdominal pain associated with nausea, vomiting, headache, and food intolerance.
Upper gastrointestinal endoscopy revealed severe gastro-esophageal reflux and
grade C esophagitis. Examination showed that he was small for his age and had
recurrent abnormal posturing, often induced by food and worsening as the day progressed. Examination did not reveal muscle hypertrophy. Abdominal tenderness
was present. When treatment of reflux disease was provided, the abnormal posturing markedly improved, confirming the diagnosis of Sandifer's syndrome.

R. Bhidayasiri, D. Tarsy, *Movement Disorders: A Video Atlas*, Current Clinical Neurology,
DOI 10.1007/978-1-60327-426-5_64, © Springer Science+Business Media New York 2012

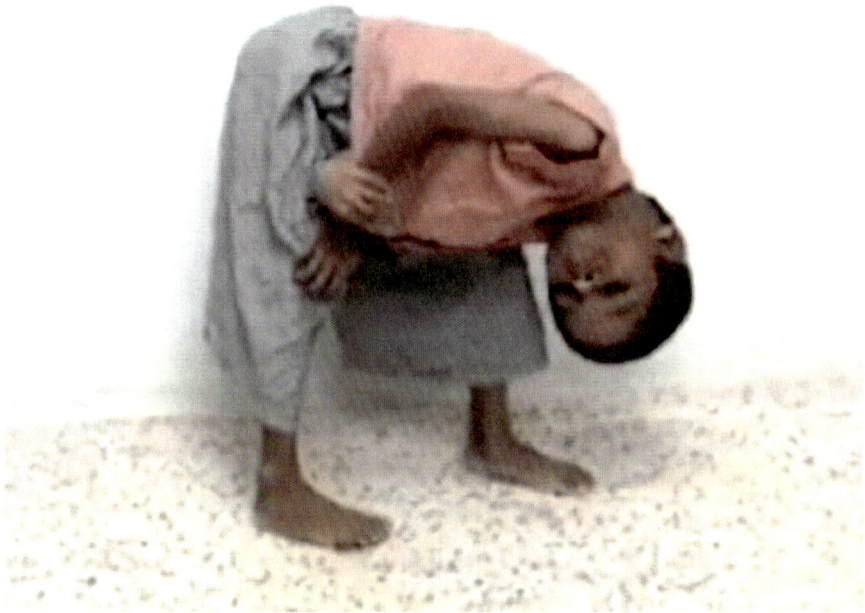

Video

The patient exhibits severe truncal flexion while standing, walking, and drawing in a crouched position with his head hanging downward. He was alert throughout the episode. (Video contribution from Dr. Asha Kishore, Sree Chitra Tirunal Institute for Medical Sciences and Technology, India.)

References

1. Kinsbourne M. Hiatus hernia with contortions of the neck. Lancet. 1964;13:1058–61.
2. Frankel EA, Shalaby TM, Orenstein SR. Sandifer syndrome: relation to abdominal wall contractions, gastroesophageal reflux, and fundoplication. Dig Dis Sci. 2006;51:635–40.

Chapter 65
Adrenoleukodystrophy

This chapter contains a video segment which can be found at the
URL: http://www.springerimages.com/Tarsy

Background

X-linked adrenoleukodystrophy (X-ALD) is an inherited disorder of peroxisomal
metabolism which is characterized by an accumulation of saturated very long chain
fatty acids. Fatty acid accumulation is associated with cerebral demyelination,
peripheral nerve abnormalities, and adrenocortical and testicular insufficiency. At
least six phenotypes have been distinguished, of which the two most frequent are
childhood-cerebral ALD and adrenomyeloneuropathy (AMN). The X-ALD gene was
identified and mapped to Xq28. Initially, only men were thought to be affected by the
disease but it is now recognized that female carriers are also at risk for X-ALD.

Childhood cerebral ALD (CCALD) is characterized by rapidly progressive cerebral demyelination. Age of onset is 3–10 years. Frequent early neurological symptoms are behavioral dysfunction, poor school performance, deterioration of vision,
and impaired auditory discrimination. The disease course usually includes seizures,
spastic tetraplegia, and dementia. In 80% of CCALD patients, cerebral MRI shows
extensive demyelination in occipital periventricular white matter. AMN is probably
the most frequent phenotype of X-ALD in the Netherlands. Onset of AMN is usually much later in life, occurring in the third or fourth decade. Neurological deficits
are primarily due to myelopathy and, to a lesser extent, peripheral neuropathy.
Patients gradually develop spastic paraparesis, often together with reduced vibration sense in the legs and urinary dysfunction. Life expectancy for those with AMN
is probably normal, unless patients also develop cerebral demyelination or adrenocortical insufficiency that is not recognized or treated. Early identification of X-ALD
is important as untreated patients with adrenocortical insufficiency require corticos-
teroid replacement. Genetic counseling should be carried out and prenatal diagnosis
is possible. Dietary supplementation with "Lorenzo's oil" (a mixture of oleic and
erucic oils) can be considered in male patients without neurological deficits, and
cerebral demyelination may be halted or reversed by bone marrow transplantation.

Case

A 14-year-old boy was referred because of progressive spasticity. There was no history of similarly affected family members. Vision was markedly impaired and limited
to finger counting. Spastic tetraplegia was present with flexion contractures in both
upper limbs. Reflexes were brisk with bilateral extensor plantar responses. There was
urinary incontinence. Brain MRI (Fig. 65.1) shows extensive periventricular white

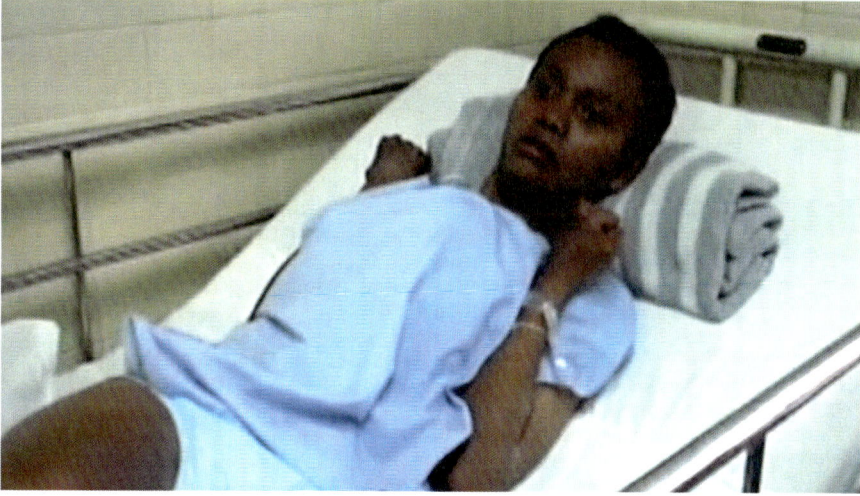

Video
This is not an example of dystonia. The examination actually shows spastic tetraplegia which is more extensive in the upper than lower limbs. There are spastic contractures in the upper limbs at the elbow and finger flexors. There is marked facial masking and absence of spontaneous movements. Vision was impaired and he was unable to cooperate for eye movement examination.

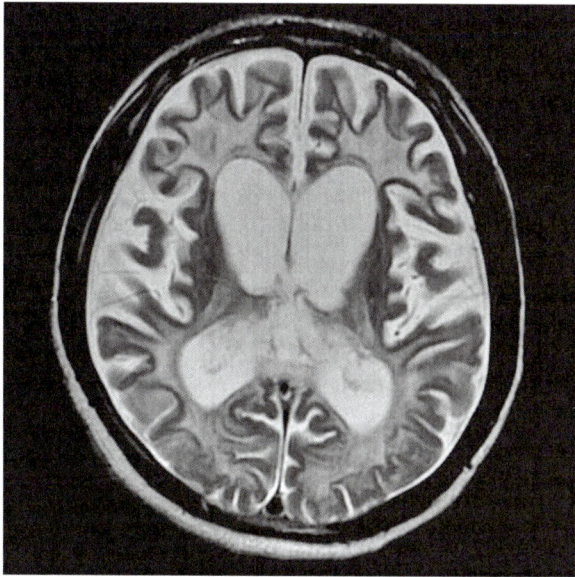

Fig. 65.1 T2-weighted brain MRI showed extensive high signal in the periventricular white matter associated with generalized brain atrophy.

matter demyelination which was predominant posteriorly. Plasma concentrations of very long chain fatty acids were highly elevated.

References

1. van Geel BM, Assies J, Wanders RJA, et al. X linked adrenoleukodystrophy: clinical presentation, diagnosis and therapy. J Neurol Neurosurg Psychiatry. 1997;63:4–14.
2. Mosser J, Douar AM, Sarde CO, et al. Putative X-linked adrenoleukodystrophy gene shares unexpected homology with ABC transporters. Nature. 1993;361:726–30.

Part IV
Choreiform Disorders

Chapter 66
Huntington's Disease

This chapter contains a video segment which can be found at the
URL: http://www.springerimages.com/Tarsy

Background

Huntington's disease (HD) is a progressive neurodegenerative disorder caused by an
expanded CAG repeat in the huntingtin gene, which encodes an abnormally long
polyglutamine repeat in the huntingtin protein. The disease is inherited in an autosomal dominant manner with age-dependent penetrance. CAG repeat lengths of 40 or
more are associated with nearly full penetrance by age 65 years. HD typically occurs
between 35 and 50 years of age. About 6% of cases have juvenile HD, defined as
disease onset before the age of 20 (see Chap. 68). In most families, age of onset tends
to be similar, but in some families the disease occurs progressively earlier in successive generations, a phenomenon called anticipation. Laboratory diagnosis is now possible with a commercially available HD gene test. Moreover, predictive genetic testing
of asymptomatic at-risk relatives should be performed in the context of family genetic
counseling. Neuroimaging usually reveals the presence of caudate atrophy.

The clinical features of HD include a triad of movement disorder, cognitive
deficit, and psychiatric/behavioral disturbances. Movement disorders include chorea and a lurching ataxia. In later stages of the disease, rigidity, dystonia, and bradykinesia often evolve while chorea improves. In addition to chorea, cognitive
impairment seems inevitable in all HD patients to a greater or lesser degree.
Although Huntington originally focused on a tendency for insanity and suicide, a
wide range of psychiatric and behavioral disturbances are known to occur. Affective
disorders are the most common of these, with depression occurring in up to 50% of
individuals. Medications used for treatment of affective disorders are therefore the
most commonly used medications in HD. The suicide rate in HD is five times that
of the general population. Psychosis is also common and, when present, is commonly associated with paranoid delusions. Antipsychotic drugs are sometimes indicated for psychiatric reasons. These may also reduce chorea but carry the risk of
causing parkinsonism. Tetrabenazine, a presynaptic dopamine depleting agent, may
be used for treatment of chorea but does not improve the gait disorder commonly
associated with HD and carries the risk of causing or aggravating depression.

Case

A 40-year-old woman presented with involuntary movements of 3 years' duration.
The movements initially involved her extremities but later extended to affect the orofacial region causing chewing movements, jaw clenching, tongue biting, and grimac-

R. Bhidayasiri, D. Tarsy, *Movement Disorders: A Video Atlas*, Current Clinical Neurology,
DOI 10.1007/978-1-60327-426-5_66, © Springer Science+Business Media New York 2012

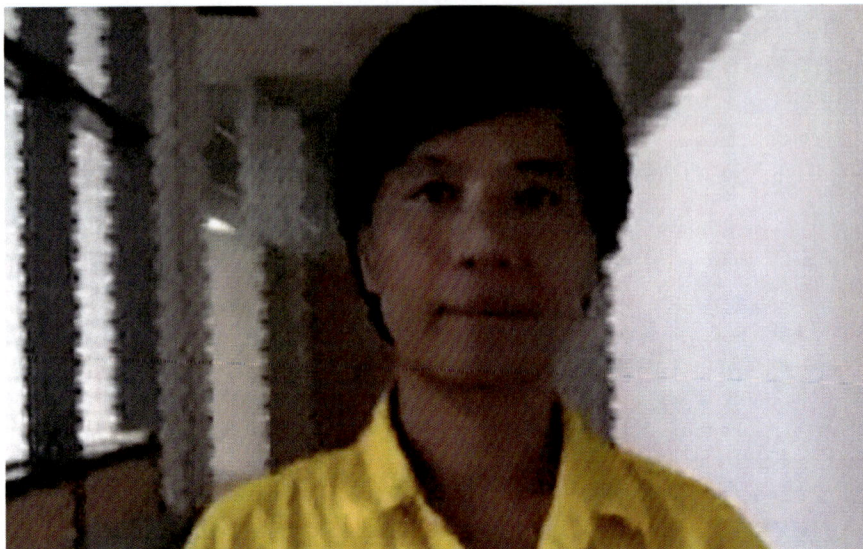

Video

Clip 1: the patient exhibits generalized chorea predominantly affecting the hands. Rocking movements of the trunk are present. Gait is slow with upper extremity chorea. Motor impersistence is present with inability to maintain tongue protrusion for longer than 10 s. *Clip 2*: mild choreiform movements of the fingers and toes are evident in her undiagnosed brother. His gait is normal except for choreiform finger movements. There is no motor impersistence of tongue protrusion.

ing. She was able to suppress these movements at times, but this led to an inner feeling of "psychic tension" that was relieved with reappearance of the movements. She lost her job as a housekeeper at age 38. Her husband reported she had become depressed and irritable with outbursts of verbal and physical abuse. Her father and paternal uncle had similar symptoms, described as being fidgety and forgetful after the age of 40 years. On examination, she had mild generalized bradykinesia with superimposed chorea affecting primarily her limbs. Facial grimacing, forceful eye blinking, and tongue protrusions were present. Relatively mild cognitive deficit was present. Tongue movements were slow with motor impersistence of tongue protrusion. Posture was stooped with a wide-based gait and tandem gait was impaired. HD genetic testing showed the HD mutation with 43 CAG repeats.

References

1. Folstein SE, Leigh RJ, Parhad IM, Folstein MF. The diagnosis of Huntington's disease. Neurology. 1986;36:1279–83.
2. HD Collaborative Group. A novel gene containing a trinucleotide repeat that is expanded and unstable on Huntington's disease chromosomes. Cell. 1993;72:971–83.
3. Guidelines for the molecular genetics predictive test in Huntington's disease. International Huntington Association (IHA) and the World Federation of Neurology (WFN) Research Group on Huntington's Chorea. Neurology 1994;44:1533–6.

Chapter 67
Late-Onset Huntington's Disease

This chapter contains a video segment which can be found at the
URL: http://www.springerimages.com/Tarsy

Background

Huntington's disease (HD) is an autosomal dominant neurodegenerative disorder
that displays marked variability in clinical manifestations and age of initial symptoms (see Chap. 66). Although average age of onset is between 40 and 50, 25% of
patients experience their initial symptoms after age 50 and onset at age 80 or above
may occur. While a preponderance of paternal transmission has been reported in
cases with juvenile-onset HD, more cases with late-onset HD seem to inherit the
affected gene from their mother. The clinical features of late-onset HD resemble
those of mid life HD, but the illness progresses more slowly and is usually less
functionally disabling. Decline in cognitive function has been found for all types of
HD, but individuals with above-average intelligence prior to onset may continue to
perform in the average range in formal testing. Slowly progressive chorea and cognitive impairment are the hallmarks of late-onset HD, and symptoms may appear to
plateau or progress very slowly for several years. The most common symptoms in
late-onset cases are mild-to-moderate chorea and cognitive impairment (100% of
the cases), dysarthria (88%), and gait disturbance (72%). Senile chorea (SC) is characterized by the presence of late-onset, generalized chorea without dementia or a
known family history of HD. It is unclear if SC is a distinct clinical entity, and several suspected SC cases have been found to have late-onset sporadic HD.

Case

A 68-year-old woman who had experienced involuntary movements since age 65
presented for treatment. Her children initially thought she was simply restless.
When the movements became more severe, she was diagnosed by her doctor as having senile chorea. There were no other similarly affected family members. The
examination revealed mild generalized chorea involving head, neck, trunk, and
limbs. Eye examination revealed mild saccadic slowing. HD genetic testing showed
40 CAG repeats in one allele.

R. Bhidayasiri, D. Tarsy, *Movement Disorders: A Video Atlas*, Current Clinical Neurology,
DOI 10.1007/978-1-60327-426-5_67, © Springer Science+Business Media New York 2012

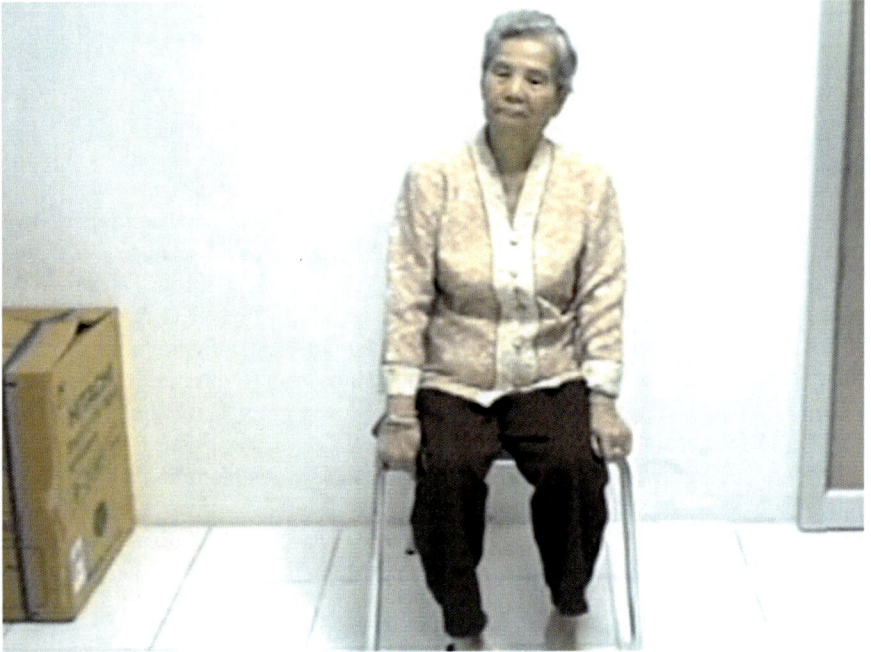

Video
The examination reveals mild generalized chorea which affects head, neck, and limbs. Mild body rocking movements are also present.

References

1. Myers RH, Sax DS, Schoenfeld M, et al. Late onset Huntington's disease. J Neurol Neurosurg Psychiatry. 1985;48:530–4.
2. James CM, Houlihan GD, Snell RG, et al. Late-onset Huntington's disease: a clinical and molecular study. Age Ageing. 1994;23:445–8.
3. Garcia Ruiz PJ, Gomez-Tortosa E, del Barrio A, et al. Senile chorea: a multicenter prospective study. Acta Neurol Scand. 1997;95:180–3.

Chapter 68
Juvenile Huntington's Disease

This chapter contains a video segment which can be found at the
URL: http://www.springerimages.com/Tarsy

Background

Huntington's disease (HD) is a rare autosomal dominant, neurodegenerative disorder
caused by a CAG DNA triplet repeat expansion in the huntingtin gene (see Chap. 66).
Onset is usually in adulthood but 1% of cases occur before age 20 and are referred
to as juvenile HD (JHD). Like HD, JHD is a progressive, autosomal dominant neurodegenerative disorder. It manifests primarily as an akinetic-rigid syndrome, with
dystonia associated with cognitive deficits and seizures. This contrasts with adult-
onset HD which usually presents with chorea and psychiatric or behavioral disturbances. At the molecular level, individuals with JHD carry large CAG expansions
in the HD gene. The length of repeat generally determines the age of onset.
Anticipation, which is earlier onset in successive generations, is more prominent
when the mutation is passed through the father. The infantile form is an extreme
form of anticipation, with the majority of patients inheriting the disease from their
father. JHD should be considered in any child with a neurodegenerative disorder
characterized by bradykinesia, rigidity, or dystonia with progressive mental deterioration and seizures, even in the absence of a positive family history.

Case

The patient is a 12-year-old right-handed girl with normal birth and early developmental milestones. Family history included an undiagnosed chronic neurological
illness in her father beginning at age 26. The patient first walked with a limp in her
left leg at age 4 which was accompanied by dysarthria. She was initially diagnosed
with hemiplegic cerebral palsy. She was relatively stable between ages 4 and 10.
However, she displayed increased difficulty walking, clumsiness in both hands, and
declining school performance. Examination showed decreased facial expression,
drooling, severe dysarthria, rigidity which was worse on the left side, bradykinesia,
and brisk reflexes with flexor plantar responses. She had mild difficulty with routine
cognitive testing and saccades were abnormally slow. There was mild chorea in
both hands and impersistence of tongue protrusion. Genetic testing showed heterozy-
gosity of the CAG repeat region on 4p16.3, with a normal allele of 17 trinucleotide
repeats and an abnormal allele of 83 repeats.

R. Bhidayasiri, D. Tarsy, *Movement Disorders: A Video Atlas*, Current Clinical Neurology,   146
DOI 10.1007/978-1-60327-426-5_68, © Springer Science+Business Media New York 2012

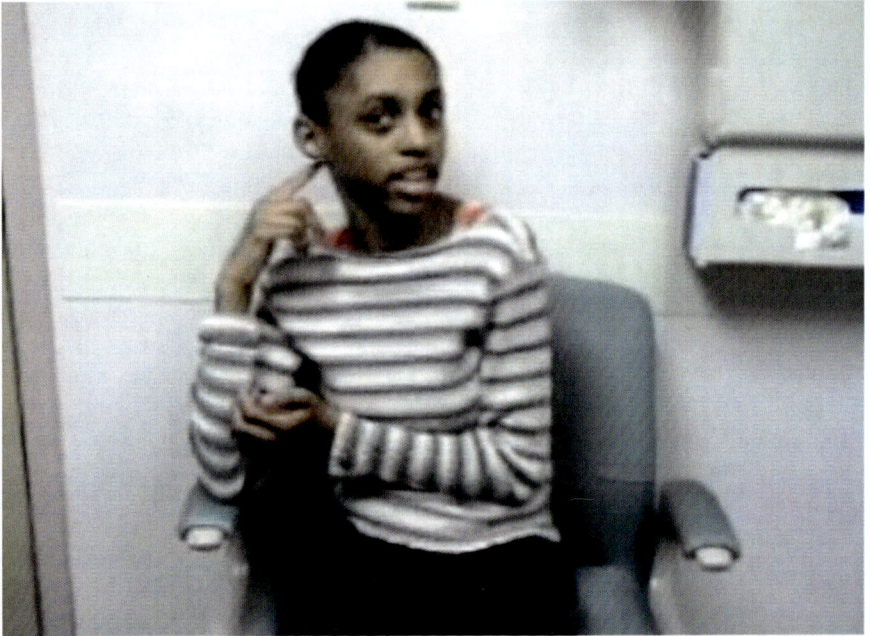

Video

The patient walks with her right arm flexed at the elbow. She walks slowly without arm swing. Facial expression is reduced, mouth is held open, and voice is hypophonic and monotonic. Cervical dystonia is present with right laterocollis and intermittent retrocollis with use of sensory tricks. Bradykinesia for finger tapping is present bilaterally. Mild chorea involves the face, tongue, and fingers, and there is impersistence of tongue protrusion.

References

1. Rasmussen A, Macias R, Yescas P, et al. Huntington disease in children: genotype-phenotype correlation. Neuropediatrics. 2000;31:190–4.
2. Ashizawa T, Wong L-J, Richards CS, et al. CAG repeat size and clinical presentation in Huntington's disease. Neurology. 1994;44:1137–43.
3. Hansotia P, Cleeland CS, Chun RWM. Juvenile Huntington's chorea. Neurology. 1968;18:217–24.

Chapter 69
Huntington's Disease-Like 2

This chapter contains a video segment which can be found at the
URL: http://www.springerimages.com/Tarsy

Background

Huntington's disease-like 2 (HDL2) is an autosomal dominant disease caused by a
trinucleotide CTG/CAG repeat expansion in the gene for junctophilin-3 located on
chromosome 16q24.3. It was initially described in a large African-American family in
the southeastern United States. Subsequent studies have shown it to be a very rare
cause of the Huntington's disease (HD) phenotype which occurs almost exclusively in
individuals of African descent. Clinically, HDL2 closely resembles HD and causes
chorea, dystonia, dysarthria, disturbed gait and balance, psychiatric symptoms, dementia, and weight loss. Onset is usually in the fourth decade with gradual progression to
death within 20 years. Similar to juvenile HD, an akinetic-rigid form without chorea
has also been described with bradykinesia, rigidity, tremor, and a frontal lobe dementia.
The neuropathology is similar to HD and includes caudate, putamen, and cortical atrophy. Diagnosis is made by gene testing. Normal CTG/CAG repeat length in the juncto-
philin-3 gene is up to 20 triplet repeats. Affected individuals with HDL2 have 41–58
triplet repeats. Similar to HD, brain MRI or CT shows caudate and cortical atrophy.
Treatment is very limited. Tetrabenazine may ameliorate the chorea but carries the risk
of aggravating bradykinesia, rigidity, and depression. Antianxiety, antidepressant, anti-
manic, and antipsychotic medications are often used as indicated.

Case

A 59-year-old Haitian woman presented with a 3-year history of involuntary movements. She was largely unaware of them, but they had become increasingly noticeable
to her daughter. These included fidgety movements of her hands and legs, rocking
movements of her head, and shifting of weight while sitting. The patient reported
unexplained falls occurring about every 2 months. She was fired from her job as a
nursing assistant a year previously because of a series of errors, following which she
became mildly depressed. Recent memory began to decline several months earlier.
Family history included her mother and brother with involuntary movements and a
sister with progressive motor deficits who became psychiatrically hospitalized. She
had two unaffected daughters and two unaffected grandchildren. Examination showed
a mild frontal dementia, continuous distal choreiform movements of her upper and
lower extremities, weight shifting while seated, and mild postural instability. There
was no bradykinesia, rigidity, or tremor. HD gene testing was normal. HDL2 gene

R. Bhidayasiri, D. Tarsy, *Movement Disorders: A Video Atlas*, Current Clinical Neurology,
DOI 10.1007/978-1-60327-426-5_69, © Springer Science+Business Media New York 2012

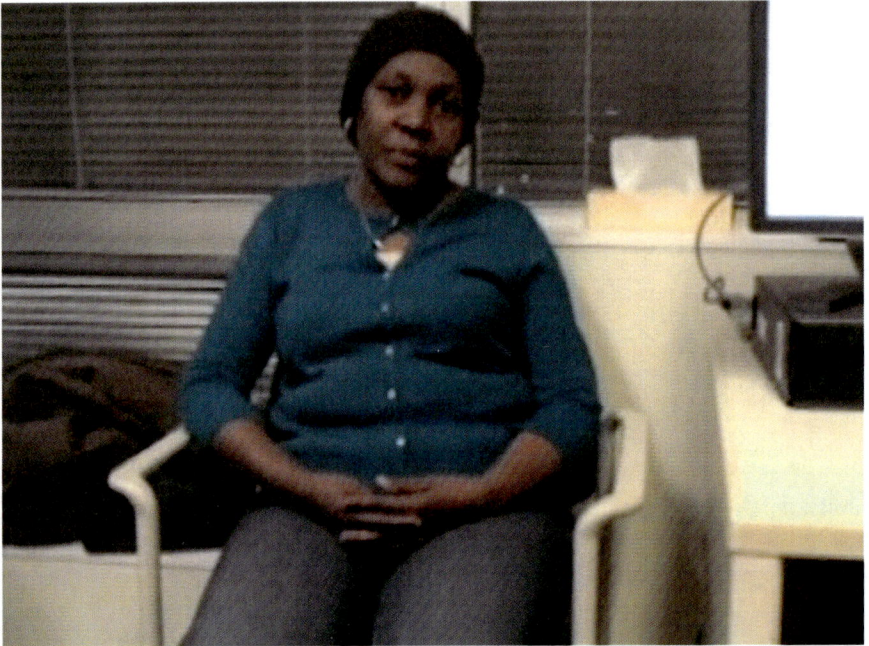

Video
The patient displays nearly continuous choreiform movements of her hands, fingers, and ankles, milder head movements, reduced facial expression, and impersistence of tongue protrusion.

testing showed 46 CAG repeats in one allele of the junctophilin gene. She was not treated with tetrabenazine because of the mild and nonintrusive nature of her chorea.

References

1. Margolis RL, O'Hearn E, Rosenblatt A. A disorder similar to Huntington's disease is associated with a novel CAG repeat expansion. Ann Neurol. 2001;50:373–80.
2. Margolis RL, Holmes SE, Rosenblatt A, et al. Huntington's disease-like 2 (HDL2) in North America and Japan. Ann Neurol. 2004;56:670–4.
3. Greenstein PE, Vonsattel JG, Margolis RL, Joseph JT. Huntington's disease-like-2 neuropathology. Mov Disord. 2007;22:1416–23.

Chapter 70
Sydenham's Chorea

This chapter contains a video segment which can be found at the
URL: http://www.springerimages.com/Tarsy

Background

Sydenham's chorea (SC) is a delayed complication of certain Aβ-hemolytic streptococcal infections and serves as a major criterion for the diagnosis of acute rheu-
matic fever. SC is characterized by chorea, muscle weakness, and a number of
neuropsychiatric symptoms. It is an antibody-mediated disorder in which patients
produce antibodies that cross-react with caudate and subthalamic nucleus neurons.
However, documented evidence of a preceding streptococcal infection is identified
in only 20–30% of cases.

Age of presentation is usually 5–15 years with a female preponderance. Chorea is
usually generalized and produces smaller amplitude and more distal involuntary
movements than those which occur in Huntington's disease. Chorea occurs at rest or
with activity and remits during sleep. The condition is generally self-limited and
remits within 16 weeks but may recur in about 20% of patients. Prognosis is good for
full recovery and treatment is therefore usually not warranted except for rare cases
associated with more severe or generalized chorea. Previously affected females are
at increased risk for developing chorea during pregnancy (chorea gravidarum) and
during sex hormone therapy. Evidence for antecedent streptococcal infection may be
derived from serially declining ASO titers and anti-DNAseB or antihyaluronidase
titers. Sedimentation rate and C-reactive protein may be elevated in acute stages of
the disease. Evidence for striatal dysfunction in Sydenham's chorea is supported by
brain MRI which, although not clinically very useful, may show lesions in the caudate and putamen in some patients and reversible striatal hypermetabolism with brain
single photon emission computed tomography during the acute illness.

Case

A 12-year-old girl who had a severe sore throat 3 months previously was referred
because of involuntary movements. Her mother stated that the abnormal movements
became so severe during the previous week that she was unable to attend school.
Her school teacher reported that she appeared to be very restless in class. Examination
revealed generalized chorea at rest and during physical activity together with
reduced attention and concentration.

R. Bhidayasiri, D. Tarsy, *Movement Disorders: A Video Atlas*, Current Clinical Neurology,   150
DOI 10.1007/978-1-60327-426-5_70, © Springer Science+Business Media New York 2012

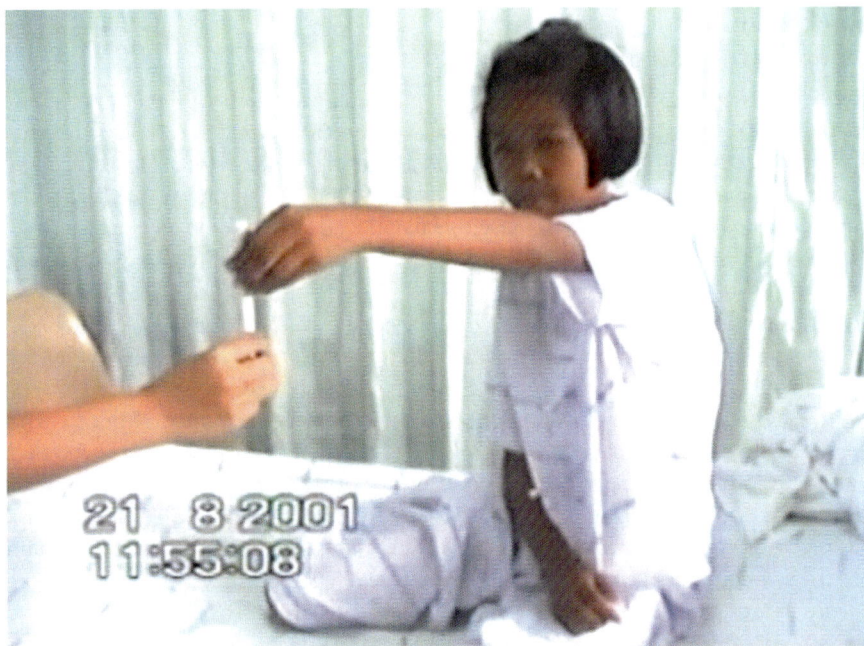

Video

The patient exhibits generalized, asymmetrical chorea which is more severe on the right side. It is more severe while extending her arms. She has difficulty maintaining continuous hand grip with her right hand. The movements are less evident while reaching for a pen. (Video contribution from Dr. Kongkiat Kulkantrakorn, Thammasat University Hospital, Thailand.)

References

1. Swedo SE. Sydenham's chorea: a model for childhood autoimmune neuropsychiatric disorder. JAMA. 1994;272:1788–91.
2. Church AJ, Cardoso F, Dale RC, et al. Anti-basal ganglia antibodies in acute and persistent Sydenham's chorea. Neurology. 2002;59:227–31.

Chapter 71
Benign Hereditary Chorea

This chapter contains a video segment which can be found at the
URL: http://www.springerimages.com/Tarsy

Background

Benign hereditary chorea (BHC) is a relatively rare autosomal dominant disorder which
produces childhood onset chorea, usually under age 5, with a stable or only slightly
progressive course. In some cases, chorea decreases in adolescence or early adulthood.
The clinical picture is apparently not identical in all families and myoclonus, dystonia,
gait disturbance, and tremor have also occasionally been present. Linkage to a region
on chromosome 14q13.1-q21.1 has been reported in several families. It is possible that
the phenotype may also be due to other yet unidentified genetic causes. Unlike
Huntington's disease (HD), BHC is not associated with behavioral changes or dementia. Brain MRI is normal. Brain technetium SPECT imaging has shown striatal and
thalamic abnormalities in a small number of patients in one family.

Case

An 83-year-old woman was referred for abnormal movements noticed by her primary care physician during a routine examination. She had been affected by these
for "as long as I can remember." They appeared to start at about age 4 when she
began school and have not increased over the years. Recently they had become
aggravated by stress. They occur at rest as well as during certain postures and mainly
affect her upper extremities. They have never interfered with any manual activities.
A deceased brother reportedly displayed identical movements from early childhood.
There was no other relevant family history. Examination showed relatively low-
amplitude choreiform movements of the arms, trunk, and large toes which increased
in amplitude and distribution during distraction maneuvers. Examination was otherwise unremarkable. Brain CT scan and DNA testing for HD were normal.

References

1. Schrag A, Quinn NP, Bhatia KP, Marsden CD. Benign hereditary chorea-entity or clinical syndrome? Mov Disord. 2000;15:80–288.
2. Breedveld GJ, Percy AK, MacDonald ME, et al. Clinical and genetic heterogeneity in benign
   hereditary chorea. Neurology. 2002;59:579–84.
3. Maahajnah M, Inbar D, Steinmetz A, et al. Benign hereditary chorea: clinical, neuroimaging,
   and genetic findings. J Child Neurol. 2007;22:1231–4.

R. Bhidayasiri, D. Tarsy, *Movement Disorders: A Video Atlas*, Current Clinical Neurology,   152
DOI 10.1007/978-1-60327-426-5_71, © Springer Science+Business Media New York 2012

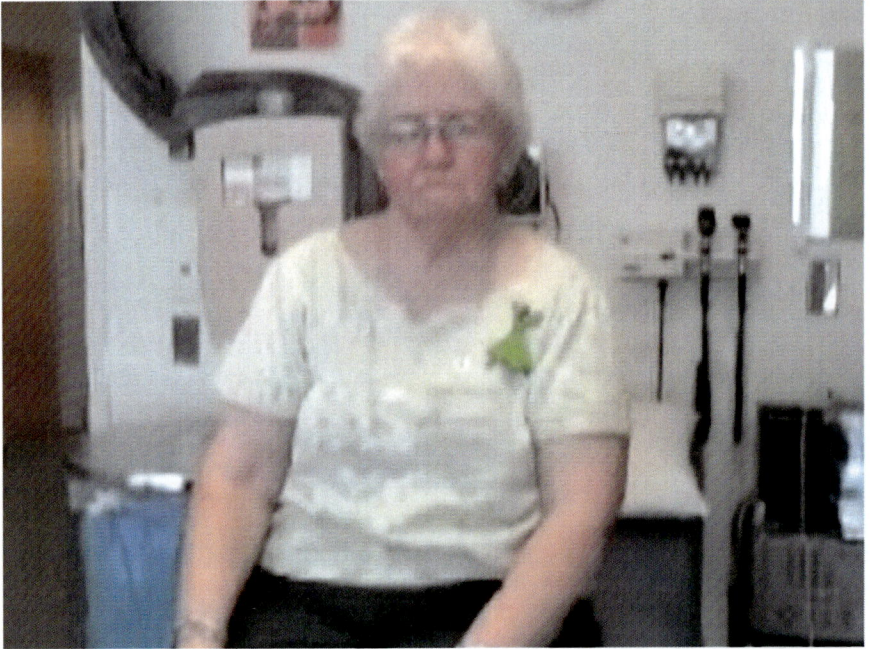

Video
The patient displays continuous low-amplitude and largely distal choreiform movement of her arms, hands, fingers, ankles, and toes.

Chapter 72
Chorea-Acanthocytosis

This chapter contains a video segment which can be found at the
URL: http://www.springerimages.com/Tarsy

Background

Chorea-acanthocytosis (ChAc) is a member of a broader group of phenotypically heterogeneous neuroacanthocytosis syndromes which include McLeod syndrome, pantothenate kinase–associated neurodegeneration (PKAN), and Huntington's disease-like
2. ChAc is an autosomal recessive disorder characterized by chorea, basal ganglia
degeneration, and acanthocytosis. Symptoms may begin at any age but often appear in
young adulthood. Tongue and lip biting are characteristic features of ChAc and may
be associated with orolingual dystonia activated by eating (see Chap. 73). Dysphagia
and dysarthria are therefore prominent. There may also be generalized chorea of varying degree, tics, stereotypies, seizures, psychiatric symptoms, and peripheral neuropathy. Brain MRI usually shows caudate and generalized atrophy. The pathology includes
prominent neuronal loss in striatum, globus pallidus, substantia nigra, and thalamus.
Most reported families display autosomal recessive inheritance but autosomal dominant, X-linked recessive, and sporadic forms have also been reported. Numerous
mutations in a chorea-acanthocytosis gene (*VPS13A* gene) on chromosome 9q21 have
been described. The McLeod phenotype is due to an X-linked recessive form of neuroacanthocytosis associated with chorea, psychiatric disorders, vocalizations, seizures, neuropathy, and liver disease but usually without lip biting or dysphagia. A
peripheral blood smear study requires special preparation and usually but not always
shows the presence of red cell acanthocytosis. Expression of chorein, a protein
encoded by the *VPS13A* gene, is reduced or absent in ChAc but not in McLeod syndrome or other forms of hereditary chorea. Treatment is directed at the specific problems which appear in each individual. Regarding management of the movement
disorders, botulinum toxin may be used for orolingual dystonia, tetrabenazine may be
used for chorea, and globus pallidus deep brain stimulation (DBS) has also been used
in several cases with mixed success.

Case

A 35-year-old man presented with a 5–10-year history of dysarthria, biting of his lips and
cheeks, involuntary tongue protrusions while eating, impaired balance, muscle weakness,
and mild cognitive changes. Examination showed lingual protrusion dystonia, hypophonia, voice tremor, and mild gait disorder. He later developed signs of mild parkinsonism.
A swallowing study showed severe oral phase dysphagia with tongue protrusions activated by attempts to chew which significantly compromised his nutrition. A diagnosis of

R. Bhidayasiri, D. Tarsy, *Movement Disorders: A Video Atlas*, Current Clinical Neurology,
DOI 10.1007/978-1-60327-426-5_72, © Springer Science+Business Media New York 2012

ChAc was made based on findings of 1–3% acanthocytosis, absence of Kell antigen, and reduced chorein. Treatment with botulinum toxin into masseter muscles and use of a mouthguard were unhelpful for tongue and cheek biting. Total tooth extraction was finally carried out which alleviated tongue and cheek biting and improved nutrition.

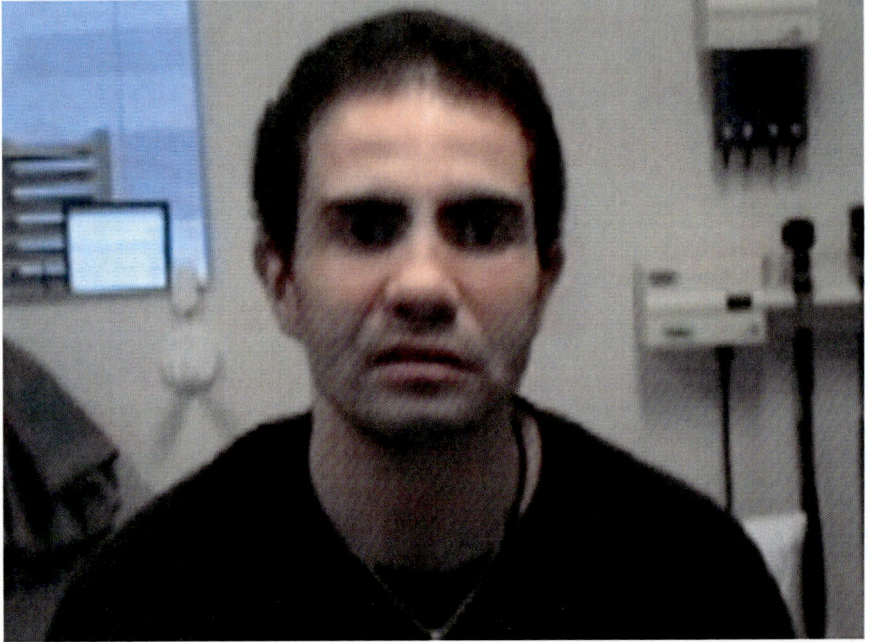

Video
The patient exhibits reduced facial expression, dysarthria, perioral tremor, and difficulty chewing due to oral phase dysphagia.

References

1. Walker RH, Jung HH, Dobson-Stone C, et al. Neurologic phenotypes associated with neuroa-canthocytosis. Neurology. 2007;68:92–8.
2. Hardie RJ, Pullon HWH, Harding AE, et al. Neuroacanthocytosis. A clinical, haematological, and pathological study of 19 cases. Brain. 1991;114:13–49.
3. Dobson-Stone C, Velayos-Baeza A, Filippone LA, et al. Chorein detection for the diagnosis of chorea-acanthocytosis. Ann Neurol. 2004;56:299–302.

Chapter 73
Chorea-Acanthocytosis with Feeding Dystonia

This chapter contains a video segment which can be found at the
URL: http://www.springerimages.com/Tarsy

Background

Chorea-acanthocytosis is the most frequent form of neuroacanthocytosis. In
addition to more generalized chorea, it frequently causes orofacial dyskinesias
associated with marked dysarthria, tongue dystonia, and dysphagia (see Chap. 72).
Protrusion tongue dystonia is particularly common in ChAc which is absent
when the mouth is at rest but occurs during orolingual manipulation of food.
Forward protrusion movements of the tongue push food out of the mouth, thereby
making chewing and swallowing very difficult. This lingual action dystonia is
highly specific for ChAc in contrast to the more spontaneous tongue protrusions
associated with other orofacial dyskinesias. Holding nonfood objects in the
mouth such as toothpicks does not provoke tongue dystonia and may be used as
a sensory trick to avoid involuntary jaw closure. The combination of masseter
and tongue protrusion dystonia commonly causes mutilations of the tongue, lips,
and cheeks and may also result in significant weight loss. Videofluoroscopy demonstrates an oral phase impaired by tongue protrusion with a relatively normal
pharyngeal phase and swallowing. Differential diagnosis of these severe orolingual dyskinesias includes Lesch-Nyhan syndrome, postanoxic states, pantothenate kinase–associated neurodegeneration, tardive dystonia, and other causes of
severe orolingual dyskinesia.

Case

A 40-year-old man presented with a 3-year history of oromandibular dyskinesia
associated with severe dyarthria and dysphagia. Examination revealed generalized
chorea and dystonia with prominent oromandibular and lingual involvement. Speech
was hypophonic, dysarthric, and frequently interrupted by lip-biting behavior.
Phonic tics, consisting of intermittent grunting sounds, also occurred. Swallowing
was difficult due to uncontrolled dystonic tongue protrusions, a phenomenon which
is called "feeding dystonia." The *VPS13A* mutation was identified by Prof. Benedikt
Bader (Ludwig-Maximilians University, Germany).

R. Bhidayasiri, D. Tarsy, *Movement Disorders: A Video Atlas*, Current Clinical Neurology,
DOI 10.1007/978-1-60327-426-5_73, © Springer Science+Business Media New York 2012

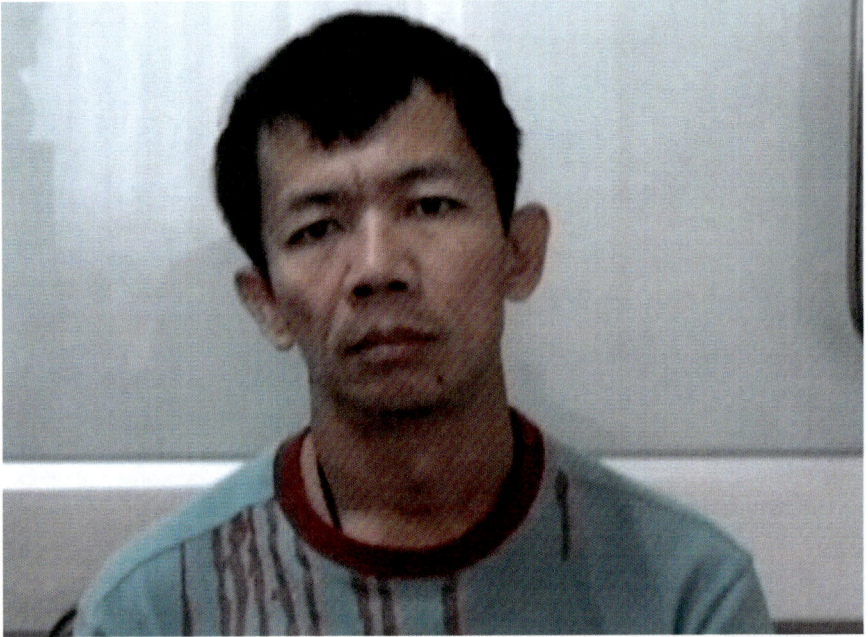

Video

This patient displays mild generalized chorea and tongue protrusion dystonia. While eating, he displays involuntary tongue movements accompanied by involuntary jaw opening. Forceful involuntary tongue protrusion is followed by voluntary retraction of the tongue. The patient tries to bypass the oral phase by pressing his lips together to close his mouth while chewing, by extending his head if the tongue protrudes, or by extending his neck so that the food falls onto the posterior portion of the tongue.

References

1. Bader B, Walker RH, Vogel M, et al. Tongue protrusion and feeding dystonia: a hallmark of chorea-acanthocytosis. Mov Disord. 2010;25:127–9.
2. Kanjanasut N, Jagota P, Bhidayasiri R. The first case report of neuroacanthocytosis in Thailand: utilization of a peripheral blood smear technique for detecting acanthocytes. Clin Neurol Neurosurg. 2010;112:541–3.

Chapter 74
Chorea-Acanthocytosis with Head Drops and Trunk Flexions

This chapter contains a video segment which can be found at the URL: http://www.springerimages.com/Tarsy

Background

Chorea-acanthocytosis (ChAc) is a rare autosomal recessive adult-onset neurodegenerative disorder due to *VPS13A* mutation of the gene encoding chorein. Clinical manifestations include mixed movement disorders, seizures, neuropathy, myopathy, autonomic features, dementia, and psychiatric disability. Because of its numerous clinical features and the availability of specialized genetic tests, clinical clues or red flags are important to assist physicians in recognizing this entity while considering other choreiform movement disorders. It has recently been suggested that flexions of the neck (presenting as head drops) as well as the trunk may be considered characteristic features of advanced ChAc.

Case

A 40-year-old man presented with a 3-year history of oromandibular dyskinesia associated with severe dyarthria and dysphagia. Examination revealed generalized chorea and dystonia with prominent oromandibular and lingual involvement. His speech was hypophonic, dysarthric, and frequently interrupted by lip-biting behavior. Phonic tics producing intermittent grunting noises were also present. Oral manipulation of food and swallowing were disturbed due to dystonic tongue protrusions, a phenomenon called "feeding dystonia" (see Chap. 73). The patient had the *VPS13A* mutation identified by Prof. Benedikt Bader (Ludwig-Maximilians University, Germany). Two years later, the patient was falling frequently and unable to sit in a chair independently. The family described his gait as a side-to-side sway of his trunk which disturbed balance.

References

1. Schneider SA, Lang AE, Moro E, et al. Characteristic head drops and axial extension in advanced chorea-acanthocytosis. Mov Disord. 2010;25:1487–91.
2. Kanjanasut N, Jagota P, Bhidayasiri R. The first case report of neuroacanthocytosis in Thailand: utilization of a peripheral blood smear technique for detecting acanthocytes. Clin Neurol Neurosurg. 2010;112:541–3.

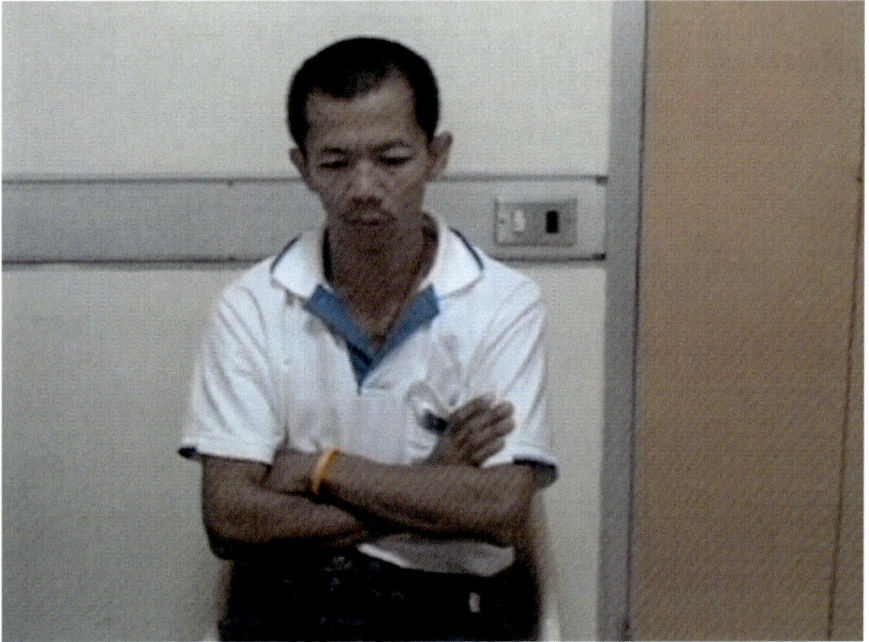

Video

The patient displays generalized chorea and tongue protrusion dystonia. While sitting, there is generalized chorea with intermittent head drops, apparently due to a sudden loss of muscle tone, together with sudden forward flexion and lateropulsion of the trunk. When asked to fold his arms, the truncal movements diminish significantly. He can also reduce the severity of head drops by putting both hands together behind his neck. Alternatively, he may stretch a towel with both hands behind his neck which also reduces the number of head drops.

Chapter 75
Hemichorea-Hemiballismus

This chapter contains a video segment which can be found at the
URL: http://www.springerimages.com/Tarsy

Background

Hemiballismus is a large amplitude, proximal, choreiform movement disorder
which affects the shoulder and upper arm and sometimes the hip and leg on one side
of the body. In some cases, the involuntary movements are smaller in amplitude and
less violent but still primarily proximal in location. In cases where milder and more
distal choreiform movements predominate, this is referred to as hemichorea. The
most common causes are ischemic or hemorrhagic lesions of the contralateral subthalamic nucleus or its connections with the globus pallidus, often among patients
with hypertension or diabetes. Small striatal infarcts may also cause hemichorea or
hemiballismus. Other lesions in this area can also cause hemiballismus including
brain abscess, demyelinating lesions, or neoplasm. Hemiballismus or hemichorea
have also been associated with nonketotic hyperglycemia where CT shows striatal
hyperintensities and MRI shows increased striatal T1 signal and reduced T2 signal
possibly due to proliferation of reactive hypertrophic astrocytes. In most cases,
symptoms cease spontaneously within weeks to months. For treatment of persistent
symptoms, dopamine receptor blocking drugs such as phenothiazines or haloperidol
and dopamine depleting drugs such as tetrabenazine are usually, but not always,
effective in reducing or eliminating the involuntary movements. Sodium valproate
and clonazepam have also occasionally been effective. In intractable cases, globus
pallidus deep brain stimulation may be considered.

Case

A 69-year-old left-handed hypertensive man developed subtle followed within several days by more obvious large amplitude proximal jerking movements of his left
shoulder and arm. The left leg became transiently involved several days later and
was severe enough to disturb his gait. Examination 10 days after onset showed intermittent proximal and distal high-frequency involuntary movements of the left shoulder and arm. CT scan showed right putamen and caudate hyperintensity while MRI
showed increased T1 signal in right putamen and caudate without evidence for
infarct or hemorrhage. Treatment with haloperidol 12 mg daily suppressed the
involuntary movements within 10 days but was associated with drug-induced parkinsonism. Subsequently careful titration with tetrabenazine successfully suppressed the hemiballismus but caused drug-induced parkinsonism (see Chap. 20).

R. Bhidayasiri, D. Tarsy, *Movement Disorders: A Video Atlas*, Current Clinical Neurology,
DOI 10.1007/978-1-60327-426-5_75, © Springer Science+Business Media New York 2012

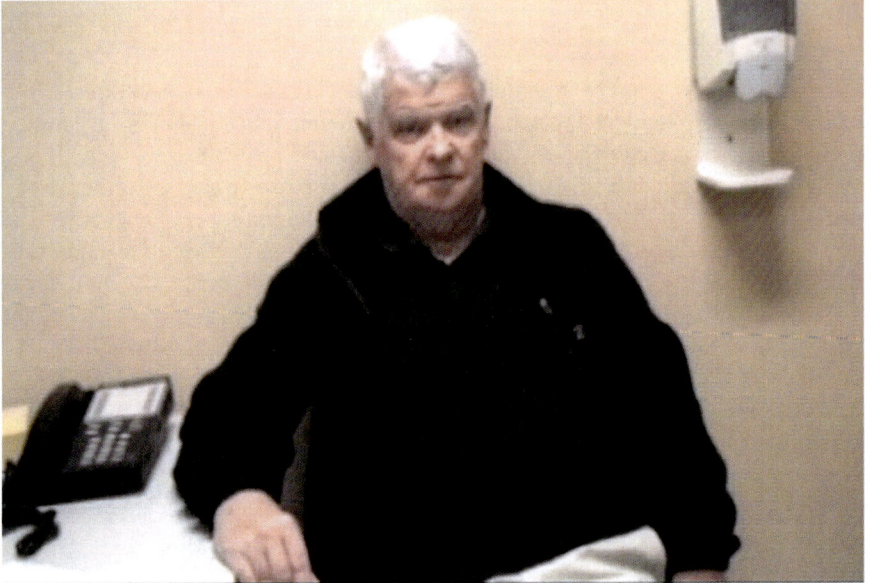

Video
The patient shows intermittent proximal and distal ballistic, dystonic, and choreiform movements involving left shoulder and wrist.

References

1. Dewey RB, Jankovic J. Hemiballismus-hemichorea clinical and pharmacologic findings in 21 patients. Arch Neurol. 1989;46:862–7.
2. Ohara S, Nakagawa S, Tabata K, Hashimoto T. Hemiballism with hyperglycemia and striatal T1-MRI hyperintensity: an autopsy report. Mov Disord. 2001;16:521–5.

Chapter 76
Chorea in Creutzfeldt-Jakob Disease

This chapter contains a video segment which can be found at the
URL: http://www.springerimages.com/Tarsy

Background

Creutzfeldt-Jakob disease (CJD) is a rare neurodegenerative disease that causes rapidly progressing dementia, myoclonus, ataxia, visual disturbance, extrapyramidal, and
pyramidal abnormalities. Approximately 90% of patients display abnormal movements, the most common of which is generalized myoclonus in advanced stages.
Several other movement disorders have been described in patients with sporadic,
familial, or new variant CJD (vCJD) including dystonia, choreoathetosis, tremor,
hemiballismus, and atypical parkinsonian features like those sometimes seen in corticobasal syndromes and progressive supranuclear palsy. The frequency of movement
disorders increases with disease duration, but these have also been reported as initial
manifestations. Myoclonus develops particularly early in patients with methionine/
methionine or methionine/valine at codon 129 of the prion protein gene and with the
scrapie variant of prion protein PrPSc type 1. Myoclonic jerks are often generalized,
relatively rhythmic, and associated with periodic sharp wave EEG activity.

Chorea has been reported in later stages of CJD and is characteristic of patients
with a definite diagnosis of vCJD. It usually appears prior to myoclonus and can be
superimposed on other abnormal movements such as dystonia. Although rare,
choreoathetosis and dyskinesia also have been reported in sporadic CJD patients
occurring more frequently and earlier when associated with the MM1 genotype.

Case

A 63-year-old English woman, a long-term resident of Thailand, presented with a
6-month history of fatigue, blurred vision, and forgetfulness. She traveled extensively, including a visit to the United Kingdom, in the 1990s. Since her return to
Thailand, she experienced fatigue and poor vision. She spoke less and sleep was
disrupted by involuntary leg movements. She also experienced episodes of confusion and disorientation and became lost in her home and while driving in familiar
neighborhoods. More recently, she developed decreased spontaneous speech and
became incapable of engaging in conversation. At her initial examination 6 months
earlier, she knew her name but was disoriented to time, place, and identification of
other people. Executive, memory processing and attention were severely impaired.
There was rigidity in the arms and legs. Spontaneous movements of the arms and
legs were accompanied by myoclonus, dysmetria, and apraxia. There was moderate
ataxia in both arms while attempting to eat.

R. Bhidayasiri, D. Tarsy, *Movement Disorders: A Video Atlas*, Current Clinical Neurology,
DOI 10.1007/978-1-60327-426-5_76, © Springer Science+Business Media New York 2012

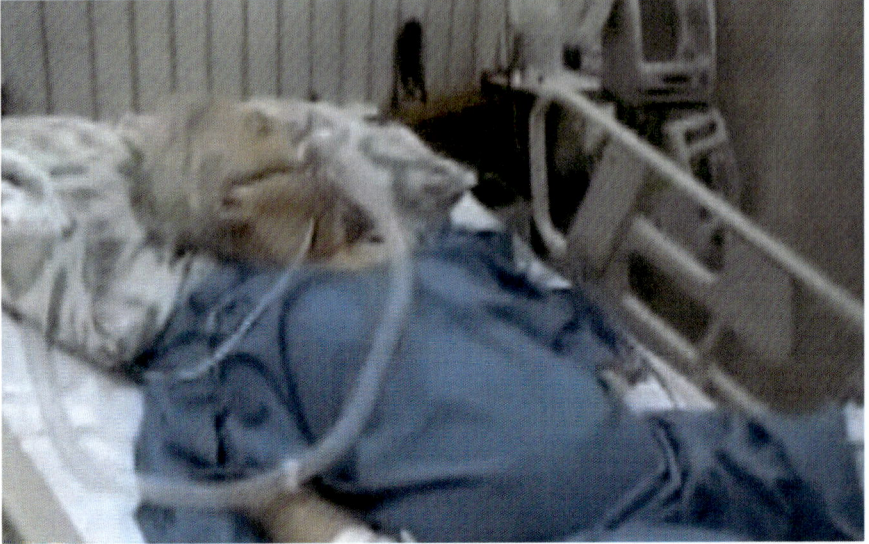

Video
The patient is intubated because of respiratory insufficiency. She exhibits generalized chorea, particularly involving both upper extremities, face, and upper trunk.

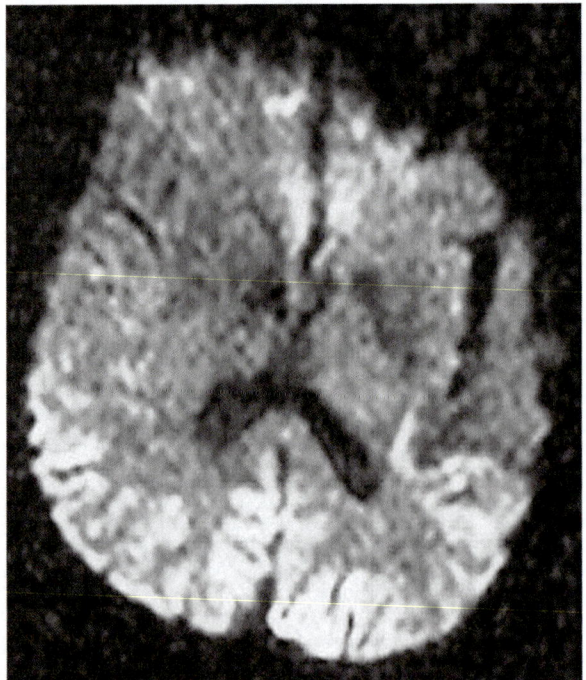

Fig. 76.1 The axial diffusion-weighted MRI showed high signal intensity in the regions of bilateral parieto-occipital lobes.

Mental status declined rapidly during the month preceding her examination and she was somnolent most of the time. Brain MRI diffusion-weighted imaging showed increased signal intensity in medial and posterior parietal and occipital cortex (Fig. 76.1). Electroencephalogram was abnormal due to diffusely slow background with periodic sharp-wave complex discharges. 14-3-3 protein was detected in the cerebrospinal fluid.

References

1. Maltete D, Guyant-Marechal L, Mihout B, et al. Movement disorders and Creutzfeldt-Jakob disease: a review. Parkinsonism Relat Dis. 2006;12:65–71.
2. Brown P, Cathala F, Castaigne P, et al. Creutzfeldt-Jakob disease: clinical analysis of consecutive series of 230 neuropathologically verified cases. Ann Neurol. 1986;20:597–602.

Chapter 77
Tardive Dyskinesia

This chapter contains a video segment which can be found at the
URL: http://www.springerimages.com/Tarsy

Background

Tardive dyskinesia (TD) refers to a movement disorder characterized by persistent
involuntary movements which appears after chronic exposure to dopamine receptor
blocking agents (DRBAs) such as antipsychotic drugs or metoclopramide. As
defined by the American Psychiatric Task Force, the diagnosis of TD requires 3
months of exposure to a DRBA, although cases occasionally appear earlier. Classical
TD is the most common persistent adverse reaction to prolonged exposure to neuroleptic medications and was the first tardive syndrome to be identified.

Typical orofacial movements include tongue protrusion, chewing (rumination),
and "bridling" (retraction of the corners of the mouth). Dyskinesia of the tongue is
characterized by protrusion or lateral tongue movements within the mouth which
may produce a bulge in the cheek, referred to as the "bonbon sign." Grimacing with
lifting or arching of the eyebrows and frowning often cause characteristic facial
expressions. Many patients exhibit repetitive flexion and extension movements of
individual fingers which resemble guitar or piano playing movements. Distal dyskinesias of the legs and repetitive stamping movements of the feet may cause walking
in place or shifting of body weight from one foot to the other. Other tardive syndromes with somewhat different clinical manifestations which have been described
include tardive dystonia, tardive akathisia, and tardive tremor.

Case

A 68-year-old woman who had been on haloperidol for more than 5 years was
referred by her dentist with a problem of chewing. She found it increasingly difficult
to keep food in her mouth because her tongue interfered with chewing and caused
frequent accidental biting of her buccal mucosa. Examination disclosed dyskinesia
of the tongue characterized by repetitive protrusion outside the mouth. Bilateral arm
rigidity was present. Her gait was slow with reduced arm swing bilaterally.

R. Bhidayasiri, D. Tarsy, *Movement Disorders: A Video Atlas*, Current Clinical Neurology,
DOI 10.1007/978-1-60327-426-5_77, © Springer Science+Business Media New York 2012

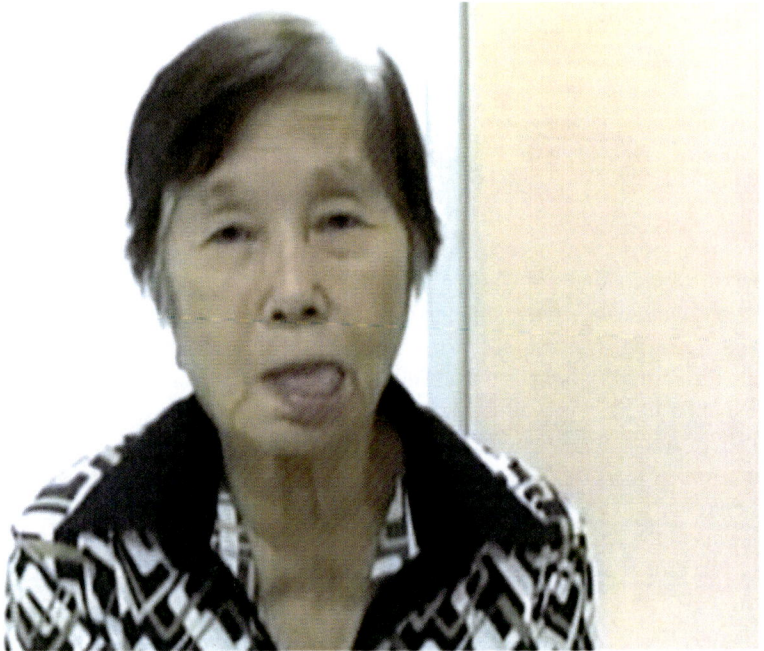

Video

The patient exhibits characteristic features of TD of the tongue with repetitive protrusion outside the mouth, retraction within the mouth, and lateral tongue movements which the patient is unable to suppress. She walks slowly with reduced arm swing bilaterally.

References

1. American Psychiatric Task Force on tardive dyskinesia. A task force report of the American Psychiatric Association. Washington D.C.: American Psychiatric Press; 1992.
2. Bhidayasiri R, Boonyawairoj S. Spectrum of tardive syndromes: clinical recognition and management. Postgrad Med J. 2011;87:132–41.
3. Fernandez HH, Friedman JH. Classification and treatment of tardive syndromes. Neurologist. 2003;9:16–27.
4. Tarsy D, Lungu C, Baldessarini RJ. In: Aminoff MJ, Boller F, Swaab DF, editors. Epidemiology of tardive dyskinesia. Handbook of clinical neurology. 3rd ed. Amsterdam: Elsevier; 2011. p. 601–16.

Chapter 78
Drug-Induced Akathisia

This chapter contains a video segment which can be found at the
URL: http://www.springerimages.com/Tarsy

Background

Akathisia refers to a state of continuous motor restlessness which, in most cases, is associated with a subjective and irresistible need to move. While sitting, akathisia produces
characteristic continuous tapping movements of the feet, repetitive movements of the
legs, and rocking movements of the trunk. In more severe cases, there is repetitive shifting of weight from 1 foot to the other and marching in place occurs while standing.
Akathisia was first described in the early twentieth century as a rare feature of a variety
of conditions including encephalitis lethargica, postencephalitic parkinsonism, myoclonus, tic disorders, and acute psychosis. However, currently, in nearly all cases akathisia
is due to drug effects. In the early 1950s, severe forms of akathisia appeared in large
numbers of patients as a side effect of antipsychotic drugs (APDs). Because of its frequent association with APD-induced acute dystonic reactions and drug-induced parkinsonism (see Chap. 20), akathisia was assumed to be an extrapyramidal disorder. However,
later descriptions emphasized the presence of strong associated feelings of internal discomfort and restlessness, raising the possibility that akathisia was an unusual response
to internal distress rather than an involuntary movement disorder.

Acute akathisia occurs shortly after treatment with dopamine receptor blocking
APDs but is often misdiagnosed as a manifestation of anxiety or psychosis. Chronic
akathisia closely resembles acute akathisia but occurs after chronic exposure to
APDs ("tardive akathisia"), is usually not accompanied by subjective need to move,
and appears to be a variant of tardive dyskinesia. Currently, most cases of acute
akathisia continue to be due to APDs but may also be caused by treatments with
serotonin reuptake inhibitors, tetrabenazine, and levodopa or levodopa withdrawal.
Differential diagnosis includes restless legs syndrome, which occurs primarily at
night and is not characterized by persistent involuntary movements, and mild choreiform disorders, which may cause fidgety limb movements and inability to keep
still (see Chap. 70). Treatment of choice for akathisia is removal of the offending
medication. Treatment with other medications such as anticholinergic drugs, beta-
blockers, or benzodiazepines is usually unsatisfactory.

Case

A 56-year-old woman developed tardive dyskinesia (TD) after receiving risperidone
for 8 years for treatment of chronic anxiety. TD was characterized by orofacial and
lingual dyskinesia and distal choreiform movement of all extremities. Attempts at

R. Bhidayasiri, D. Tarsy, *Movement Disorders: A Video Atlas*, Current Clinical Neurology,
DOI 10.1007/978-1-60327-426-5_78, © Springer Science+Business Media New York 2012

treatment with a variety of medications including benzodiazepines, Clozaril, quetia-pine, reserpine, levetiracetam, aripiprazole, and haloperidol were all either ineffec-tive or produced adverse effects. Tetrabenazine (TBZ), titrated to 125 mg/day, finally suppressed the dyskinesias but caused severe subjective and objective akath-isia, which was different in appearance from her TD, and cleared when it was dis-continued. This was followed by prompt return of all signs of TD. Bilateral globus pallidus deep brain stimulation was performed which produced nearly complete relief of dyskinesia.

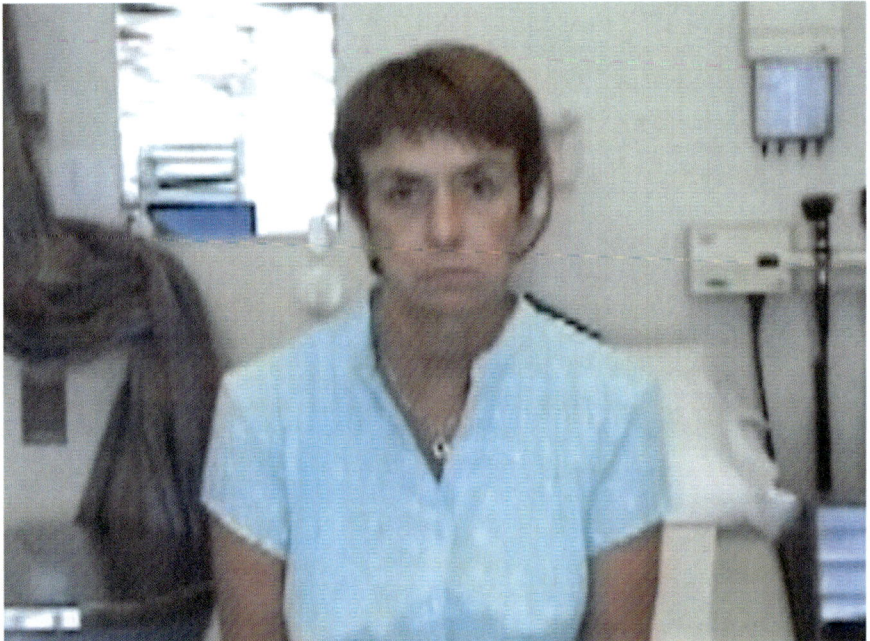

Video

Clip 1: patient is off APDs and displays continuous orofacial dyskinesia and choreoathetotic move-ments of her distal extremities. She has had recent left carpal tunnel surgery. *Clip 2*: patient is now on TBZ and is no longer displaying orofacial or lower limb dyskinesia. Instead, she shows signs of typical akathisia with continuous tapping movements of her legs while seated and standing. She describes a strong need to move which was not present prior to the use of TBZ. She has now had recent right carpal tunnel surgery (Video contribution from Dr. Ludy Shih, Beth Israel Deaconess Medical Center, Boston).

References

1. Tarsy D. Akathisia. In: Joseph AB, Young RR, editors. Movement disorders in neurology and neuropsychiatry. Boston: Blackwell; 1992. p. 88–99.
2. Stahl SM. Akathisia and tardive dyskinesia: changing concepts. Arch Gen Psychiatry. 1985; 42:915–7.

Chapter 79
Edentulous Dyskinesia

This chapter contains a video segment which can be found at the URL: http://www.springerimages.com/Tarsy

Background

Edentulous dyskinesia (ED) is characterized by excessive, aimless, stereotyped movements of the jaw, mouth, and tongue which occur in elderly edentulous individuals. It occurs in 7–13% of edentulous subjects either with or without dental prostheses. Some individuals are referred to as having "spontaneous orofacial dyskinesia of the elderly." The mechanism responsible for ED is poorly understood, but it has been suggested that malocclusion and reduced sensory feedback from oral structures may play a role since the loss of sensory nerve endings in periodontal ligaments following multiple tooth extractions may cause proprioceptive defects.

ED has been commonly confused with oral forms of tardive dyskinesia (TD) because the abnormal movements of the lips, tongue, and jaw may have a similar appearance. However, ED can be distinguished from oral TD based on its orodental and motor features. Unlike TD, excessive movements in ED are limited to the oral or facial region, and the tongue does not usually show dystonic movements when the mouth is open. ED also does not usually produce prominent, protrusion tongue movements such as the "fly-catcher tongue" often observed in TD. ED is also not associated with the sustained muscular contractions which cause prolonged spasms of the jaw which occur in oromandibular dystonia.

Case

An 82-year-old woman was not aware of abnormal oral movements and denied any history of exposure to antipsychotic drugs. She reported problems with ill-fitting dentures and dental pain when chewing for several years. She had several tooth extractions during the previous year. Examination revealed poor oral hygiene with numerous dental caries. There was significant malocclusion. The oral movements consisted of intermittent side-to-side movements of the jaw. Tongue or facial dyskinesia was not present.

R. Bhidayasiri, D. Tarsy, *Movement Disorders: A Video Atlas*, Current Clinical Neurology, DOI 10.1007/978-1-60327-426-5_79, © Springer Science+Business Media New York 2012

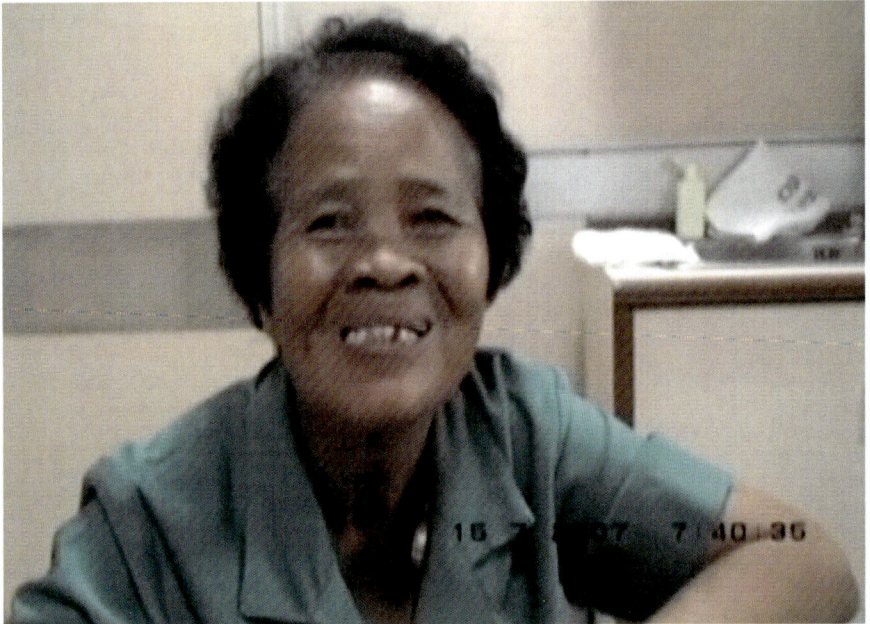

Video
The patient exhibits intermittent lateral movements of the jaw associated with malocclusion. The
patient is unaware of the abnormal movements.

References

1. Koller WC. Edentulous orodyskinesia. Ann Neurol. 1983;13:97–9.
2. Blanchet PJ, Popovici R, Guitard F, et al. Pain and denture condition in edentulous orodyskinesia: Comparisons with tardive dyskinesia and control subjects. Mov Disord. 2008;23:1837–42.

Chapter 80
Painful Legs and Moving Toes

This chapter contains a video segment which can be found at the
URL: http://www.springerimages.com/Tarsy

Background

Painful legs and moving toes (PLMT) is a very uncommon disorder in which patients
experience pain in their legs together with continuous involuntary movements of
their toes. Pain is usually the first and predominant symptom. The pain is typically
deeply seated and is usually described as a severe aching, pulling, or crushing sensation in the lower legs. Persistent toe movements may not be reported but are evident
on examination and consist of flexion-extension or abduction-adduction fanning
movements with a frequency of 1–2 Hz. In severe cases, more proximal leg movements may also be present. Patients can usually suppress the toe movements for
short periods of time, but they typically promptly return within moments. Symptoms
are usually bilateral but may occasionally present unilaterally. Much less common
variants of PLMT have been reported such as painful hand and moving fingers and
painless legs and moving toes. In most cases, symptoms appear on a background of
lumbosacral radiculopathy, peripheral neuropathy, or lower extremity injury which,
together with the character of the pain, suggests that PLMT may be a variant of
complex regional pain syndrome. PLMT is often mistaken for restless legs syndrome but differs in that the toe movements are involuntary while in restless legs
syndrome any associated leg movements are voluntary attempts to relieve leg discomfort. Response to various treatments has been variable but usually disappointing
and has included sympathetic blockade, guanethidine blocks, transcutaneous nerve
stimulation, anticonvulsants, and antidepressants.

Case

A 63-year-old woman experienced pain and hypersensitivity to touch of both feet
followed within several months by involuntary movements of her toes present only
when seated or lying down. This occurred on a background of type 2 diabetes and
liver cirrhosis. Symptoms persisted for the next 4 years. Examination showed continuous flexion-extension movements of the toes while standing, seated, or reclining. Vibration, position, and light touch were reduced in the feet but there was no
allodynia. Ankle reflexes were absent. Pain was reasonably well controlled on a
combination of gabapentin and duloxetine, but disturbing toe movements persisted
unchanged without response to clonazepam or botulinum toxin injections into the
flexors and extensors of the toes.

R. Bhidayasiri, D. Tarsy, *Movement Disorders: A Video Atlas*, Current Clinical Neurology,
DOI 10.1007/978-1-60327-426-5_80, © Springer Science+Business Media New York 2012

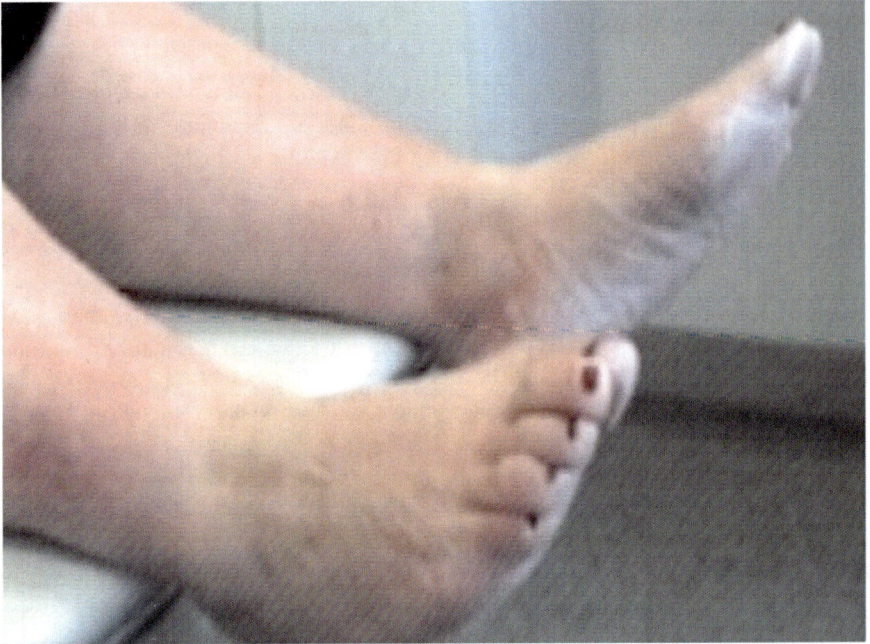

Video
While reclining, the patient displays continuous flexion-extension movements of the toes.

References

1. Spillane JD, Nathan PW, Kelly RE, Marsden CD. Painful legs and moving toes. Brain. 1971;94:541–56.
2. Dressler D, Thompson PD, Gledhill RF, Marsden CD. The syndrome of painful legs and moving toes. Mov Disord. 1994;9:13–21.
3. Alvarez MV, Driver-Dunckley E, Caviness JN, et al. Case series of painful legs and moving toes: clinical and electrophysiological observations. Mov Disord. 2008;23:2062–6.

Chapter 81
"Postpump" Chorea

This chapter contains a video segment which can be found at the
URL: http://www.springerimages.com/Tarsy

Background

Postpump chorea is characterized by choreoathetoid movements which sometimes
appear in children following cardiopulmonary bypass surgery, usually within 2
weeks of surgery. Approximately 1% of children who have cardiac surgery develop
this syndrome. The mean age of affected individuals is 8–34 months. Risk factors
include deep hypothermia and circulatory arrest. This syndrome is often later associated with developmental delay and neurological deficits ranging from mild learn-
ing disabilities to progressive hypotonia with obtundation. Chorea can be transient
or persistent. Neuroimaging usually reveals brain atrophy without focal abnormalities. The mechanism for this syndrome is not entirely clear, but the literature suggests it may be the result of microembolic phenomena of air, fat, shards of
polyvinylchloride tubing, antifoaming agents, and/or platelet fibrin aggregates
accumulated during surgery.

Case

A 9-month-old girl was admitted to hospital for correction of tetralogy of Fallot.
She had normal preoperative growth and development. She was placed into deep
hypothermia during surgery. There were no perioperative complications, and the
first 5 postoperative days were uneventful. On the sixth postoperative day, the patient
became very irritable. She cried constantly and displayed choreiform movements of
the face, trunk, and extremities. Truncal hypotonia was also present. Brain MRI was
unremarkable.

References

1. Medlock MD, Cruse RS, Winek SJ, et al. A 10-year experience with postpump chorea. Ann
   Neurol. 1993;34:820–6.
2. Wong PC, Barlow CF, Pr H, et al. Factors associated with choreoathetosis after cardiopulmonary bypass in children with congenital heart disease. Circulation. 1992;86:118–26.

R. Bhidayasiri, D. Tarsy, *Movement Disorders: A Video Atlas*, Current Clinical Neurology,   174
DOI 10.1007/978-1-60327-426-5_81, © Springer Science+Business Media New York 2012

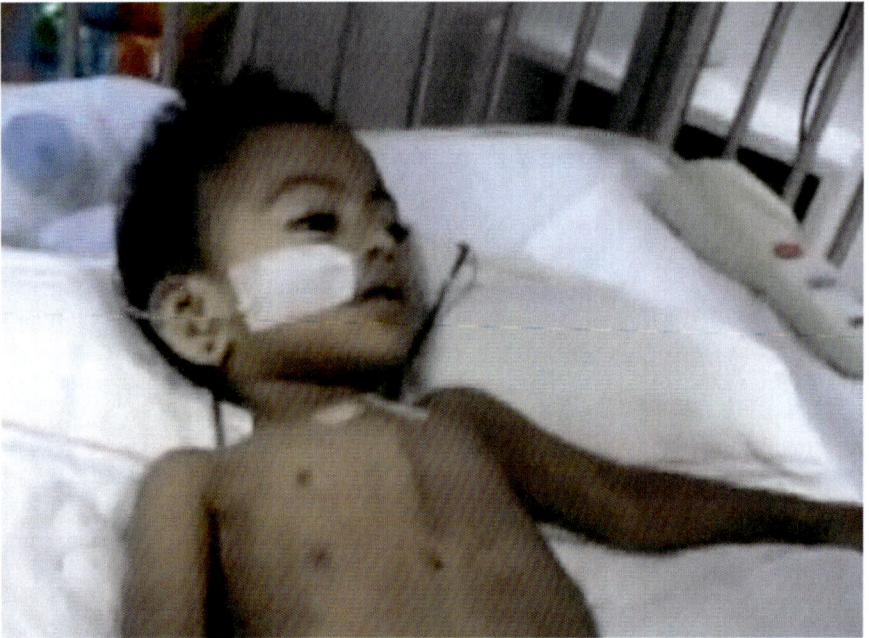

Video

The child is irritable and has choreiform movements of the face and tongue protrusions with less chorea in the extremities. Occasionally, there are ballistic movements of the left arm. Fine tremulous movements were observed in the extremities. She has severe truncal hypotonia.

Chapter 82
Belly Dancer's Dyskinesia

This chapter contains a video segment which can be found at the
URL: http://www.springerimages.com/Tarsy

Background

The term "belly dancer's dyskinesia" refers to a form of focal dyskinesia affecting
the abdominal wall. The clinical characteristics of this unusual dyskinesia are somewhat variable but usually consist of writhing movements and contractions of the
abdominal muscles. These movements cannot be voluntarily suppressed but may be
influenced by respiratory maneuvers. Onset is usually gradual and has sometimes
occurred following local trauma or abdominal surgical procedures. It is also a common manifestation of tardive dyskinesia due to long-term use of dopamine receptor
blocking agents. It may also occur in the setting of a psychogenic movement disorder. Investigations such as spinal and abdominal imaging usually fail to reveal any
local abnormalities to explain the movement disorder. Prognosis is unfavorable as
there is no known effective treatment. The clinical course may therefore be long-
lasting or permanent.

Case

A 15-year-old girl presented with involuntary movements of the abdominal wall
which she had been experiencing for 6 months. Medical history included a mild
back injury in a motor vehicle accident without any apparent sequelae. There was
no exposure to antipsychotic drugs or metoclopramide. She had been aware of intermittent involuntary abdominal contractions for several months. She complained of
mild discomfort around the navel but was not very distressed by the movements. On
examination, there were continuous, slow, contorting movements of the abdominal
wall which produced slow displacement of the umbilicus in several directions. The
movements occasionally alternated from the left to the right side, producing a side-
to-side motion of the abdomen. The movements were not relieved during deep
inspiration or breath-holding. There were no other abnormal neurological signs, and
the rest of the physical examination was normal.

R. Bhidayasiri, D. Tarsy, *Movement Disorders: A Video Atlas*, Current Clinical Neurology,
DOI 10.1007/978-1-60327-426-5_82, © Springer Science+Business Media New York 2012

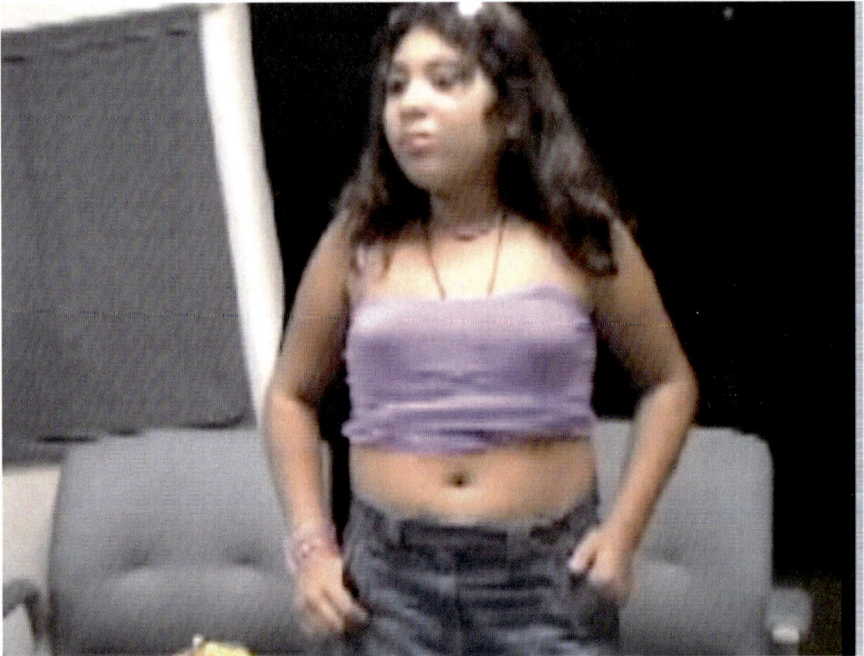

Video

Slow contorting and writhing movements of the anterior abdominal wall are evident, resulting in displacement of the umbilicus in various directions. The patient occasionally voluntarily shrugged her shoulders in response to her abdominal discomfort.

References

1. Iliceto G, Thompson PD, Day BL, et al. Diaphragmatic flutter, the moving umbilicus syndrome, and "belly dancer's" dyskinesia. Mov Disord. 1990;5:15–22.
2. Linazasoro G, Blercom NV, Lasa A, et al. Etiological and therapeutical observations in a case of belly dancer's dyskinesia. Mov Disord. 2005;20:251–3.
3. Caviness JN, Gabellini A, Kneebone CS, et al. Unusual focal dyskinesias: the ears, the shoulders, the back and the abdomen. Mov Disord. 1994;9:531–8.

Chapter 83
Pseudoathetosis

This chapter contains a video segment which can be found at the URL: http://www.springerimages.com/Tarsy

Background

Athetosis refers to continuous involuntary movements of the distal extremities, usually involving the digits, hands, and feet. Pseudoathetosis is characterized by very similar involuntary, slow, writing movements of the digits and distal extremities occurring with the eyes closed which closely resembles athetosis. This disorder is caused by impaired proprioception, while in athetosis there is no sensory loss. The lesion responsible for pseudoathetosis may be located anywhere in sensory pathways between peripheral nerve and parietal cortex, including especially posterior columns in cervical cord and thalamus. Most patients are unaware of abnormal movements when their eyes are closed. Opening or closing the eyes may have an inconsistent effect on the severity of the movements. While the exact mechanism of pseudoathetosis is uncertain, it is hypothesized that it occurs because of a failure to process limb proprioceptive information in the striatum. Therefore, both choreoathetosis and pseudoathetosis may be manifestations of a failure of the striatum to properly integrate cortical motor and sensory inputs.

Case

A 65-year-old woman presented with severe headaches and neck pain. She complained that both legs were weak and reported she was having repeated falls. Examination revealed that both legs were spastic and hyperreflexic. Muscle strength was normal in proximal muscles of both arms and legs. Plantar responses were extensor. With eyes closed, there were slow, writhing, vermicular movements of all fingers and the wrists which the patient was unaware of. Position and vibration sense were absent in the feet, markedly reduced in the legs and moderately reduced in the hands. Gait was ataxic and she required assistance to walk. Brain MRI T1 weighted images with gadolinium showed an enhancing cerebellar mass compressing the brainstem (Fig. 83.1).

R. Bhidayasiri, D. Tarsy, *Movement Disorders: A Video Atlas*, Current Clinical Neurology, DOI 10.1007/978-1-60327-426-5_83, © Springer Science+Business Media New York 2012

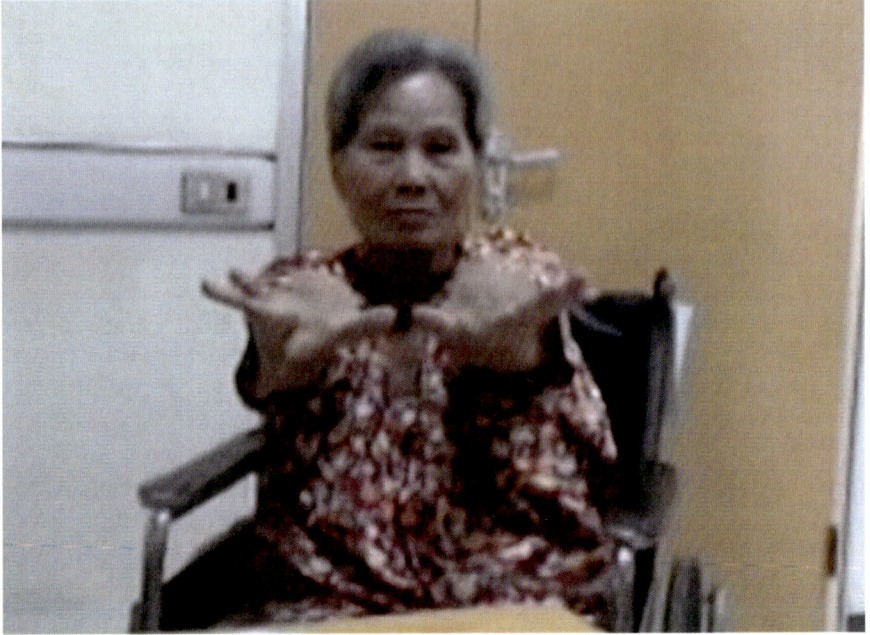

Video

The patient exhibits continuous choreoathetotic movements of the fingers of both hands. Both index fingers display repeated dystonic postures. When she closes her eyes, the involuntary movements appear to worsen. Her gait is unsteady on a narrow base, and she requires assistance to walk.

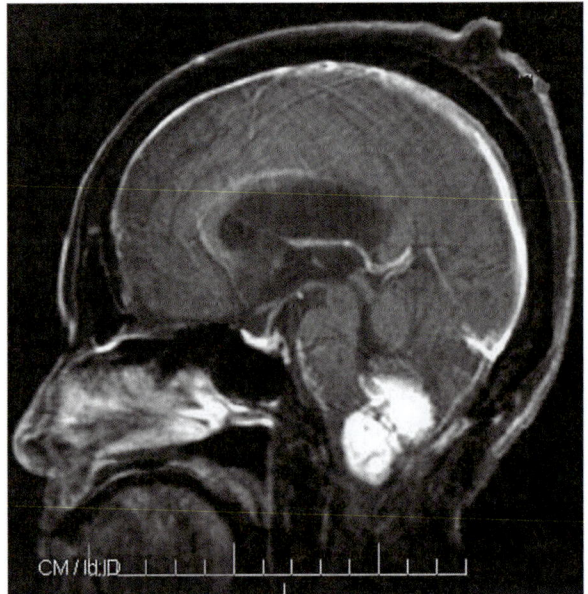

Fig. 83.1 Sagittal postgadolinium T1-weighted brain MRI showed an enhancing round mass within the cerebellum compressing lower brainstem and upper spinal cord.

References

1. Sharp FA, Rando TA, Greenberg SA, et al. Pseudochoreoathetosis: movements associated with loss of proprioception. Arch Neurol. 1994;51:1103–9.
2. Spitz M, Machado AAC, Carvalho RC, et al. Pseudoathetosis: report of three patients. Mov Disord. 2006;21:1520–2.
3. Ghika J, Bogousslavsky J. Spinal pseudoathetosis A rare, forgotten syndrome, with a review of old and recent descriptions. Neurology. 1997;49:432–7.

Part V
Myoclonus

Chapter 84
Brainstem Myoclonus

This chapter contains a video segment which can be found at the
URL: http://www.springerimages.com/Tarsy

Background

Two types of brainstem myoclonus are recognized: (1) exaggerated startle myoclonus and (2) reticular reflex myoclonus. Brainstem myoclonus is generated mainly in
the reticular formation which lies close to the accessory nerve nuclei. Clinically, the
muscle jerks of reticular reflex myoclonus are usually generalized with proximal
more than distal and flexor more than extensor predominance. Voluntary action and
sensory stimulation may increase the muscle jerks. Neurophysiologically, the first
recruited muscle which jerks is the sternocleidomastoid or trapezius muscle. The
myoclonic discharge then travels down the spinal cord and up the brainstem.

A variant of reticular reflex myoclonus, carotid brainstem reflex myoclonus, has
been described in a comatose patient after acute anoxia. This patient developed
bilaterally synchronous, periodic myoclonic jerks which were most prominent in
the upper limbs. Electrophysiologic studies showed that the myoclonus jerks correlated in timing and size with arterial pulses and were suppressed by massage over
the carotid sinus.

Case

A 65-year-old woman was comatose due to a pontine hemorrhage. She had intermittent jerks of the upper limbs bilaterally. The jerks mainly involved the shoulders and
proximal upper limbs on each side. They occurred both spontaneously and after
stimulation. Reticular reflex myoclonus was suspected based on its predilection for
accessory nerve innervated muscles and the anatomical location of the pontine
hemorrhage.

References

1. Hallett M. Neurophysiology of brainstem myoclonus. Adv Neurol. 2002;89:99–102.
2. Hanakawa T, Hashimoto S, Iga K, et al. Carotid brainstem reflex myoclonus after hypoxic brain
damage. J Neurol Neurosurg Psychiatry. 2000;69:672–4.

R. Bhidayasiri, D. Tarsy, *Movement Disorders: A Video Atlas*, Current Clinical Neurology,   182
DOI 10.1007/978-1-60327-426-5_84, © Springer Science+Business Media New York 2012

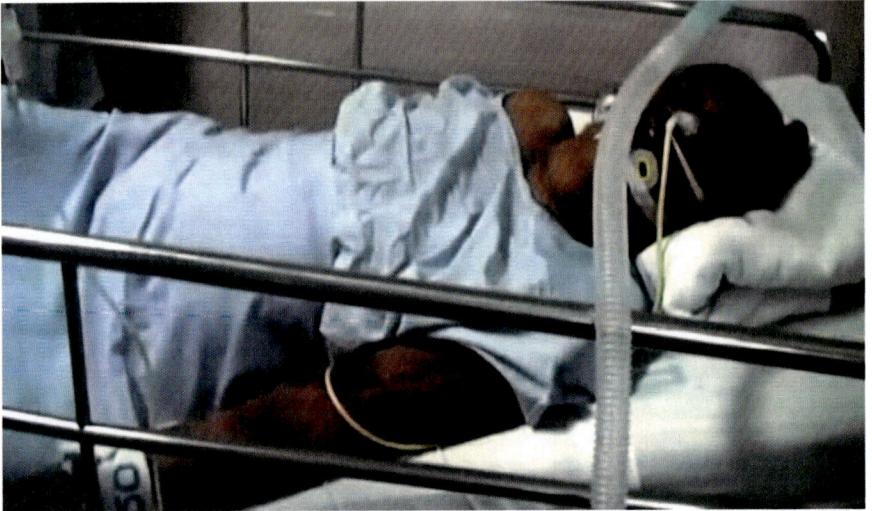

Video

The patient exhibits myoclonic jerks involving her shoulders and proximal portions of her upper extremities bilaterally. The jerks occur spontaneously but are more frequent after pressure over the sternum.

Chapter 85
Palatal Myoclonus

This chapter contains a video segment which can be found at the
URL: http://www.springerimages.com/Tarsy

Background

Palatal myoclonus (PM), also known as palatal tremor, is a rare disorder which
causes low-frequency 1–3 Hz contractions of the uvula and soft palate. Secondary
PM most commonly occurs secondary to a lesion in the brainstem or cerebellum
within Mollaret's triangle which comprises the cerebellar dentate nucleus, red
nucleus, central tegmental tract, and inferior olivary nucleus. There is sometimes
associated myoclonus of the face, eye muscles, tongue, or larynx. Secondary PM is
due to rhythmic contractions of the levator veli palatine muscle. Primary or essential
PM is less common, occurs in the absence of an identifiable lesion, is usually isolated, produces audible ear clicking, and is usually absent during sleep. Symptoms
of PM are usually mild and limited to ear clicking but severe cases may disturb
speaking or swallowing. PM may not be continuous, may cease during phonation or
swallowing, and may be inhibited under voluntary control. Treatment with anticonvulsants or anticholinergic drugs is only sometimes helpful, while botulinum toxin
injections into the involved muscles are usually very effective.

Case

A 41-year-old woman with a 14-year history of cervical dystonia developed intermittent ear clicking and a "rising" sensation in her throat. Examination showed rhythmic
PM with occasional brief interruptions which could be briefly interrupted voluntarily.
There were no other involuntary movements except for mild right-sided rotational
torticollis which was responsive to botulinum toxin and had been unchanged for
14 years. Brain MRI was normal. The PM was felt to be unrelated to antecedent cervical dystonia and a diagnosis of essential PM was made. Clonazepam and sertraline
were unhelpful, and she declined palatal botulinum toxin injections. Palatal myoclonus has become less symptomatic but has persisted unchanged over the next 6 years.

References

1. Deuschl G, Mischke G, Schenck E, Schulte-Monting J, Lucking CH. Symptomatic and essential rhythmic palatal myoclonus. Brain. 1990;113:1645–72.
2. Cho JW, Chu K, Jeon BS. Case of essential palatal tremor: atypical features and remarkable
benefit from botulinum toxin injection. Mov Disord. 2001;16:779–82.

R. Bhidayasiri, D. Tarsy, *Movement Disorders: A Video Atlas*, Current Clinical Neurology,
DOI 10.1007/978-1-60327-426-5_85, © Springer Science+Business Media New York 2012

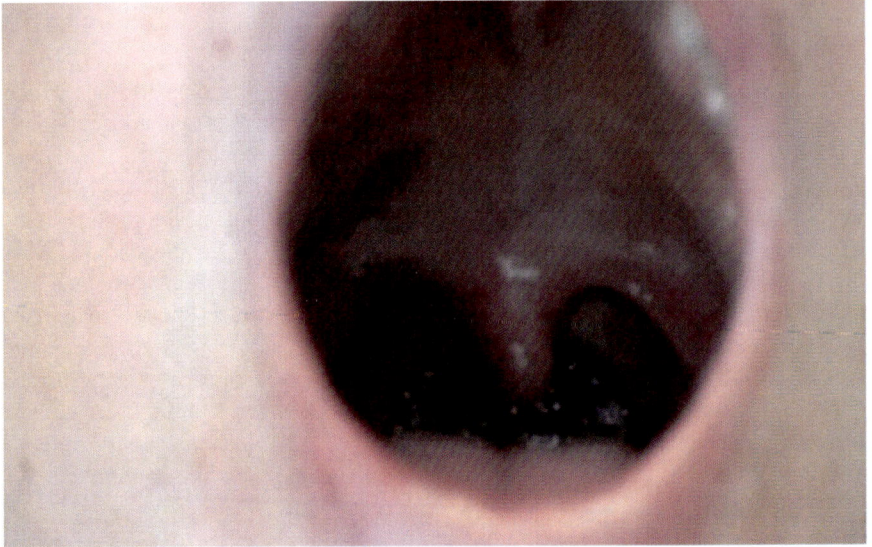

Video
Intraoral video shows irregular low-frequency (about 2 Hz) PM.

Chapter 86
Posthypoxic Myoclonus

This chapter contains a video segment which can be found at the
URL: http://www.springerimages.com/Tarsy

Background

Posthypoxic myoclonus (PHM) is characterized by severe action myoclonus associated with cerebellar ataxia, postural lapses, gait disturbances, and grand mal seizures. PHM develops following episodes of hypoxic-ischemia caused by cardiac
arrest or airway obstruction. Respiratory arrest experienced during an acute asthma
attack is a common precipitating event which is followed in frequency by anesthetic
and surgical accidents. Acute PHM typically occurs within 24 h after a hypoxic
episode and is characterized by severe, generalized myoclonic jerks (typically violent flexion movements) in patients who are deeply comatose. When these persist
for over 30 min or occur during most of the first post-resuscitation day, some clinicians consider the abnormal movements to represent myoclonic status epilepticus.
Chronic PM, known as Lance-Adams syndrome, typically begins within several
days to weeks after hypoxic brain injury. Clinical features include positive myoclonic jerks precipitated by any attempts to move, particularly movements requiring
coordination or dexterity such as goal-directed movements. Myoclonic jerks tend to
improve or even disappear when the patient relaxes but may be stimulus-sensitive
and may be triggered by startle or strong emotion. Other associated neurological
signs include dysmetria, gait ataxia, dysarthria, and intention tremor.

Posthypoxic myoclonus is believed to arise either cortically or subcortically, although
both forms may coexist. Cortical myoclonus originates in sensory-motor cortex, involves
the limbs or face, and is triggered by activity or goal-directed movements. Less commonly PM is the result of subcortical myoclonus, also known as reticular reflex myoclonus, which originates from the brainstem and produces proximal, generalized jerks that
are often stimulus-sensitive (see Chap. 84). Neurological deficits often gradually resolve
over time, leaving only persistent action myoclonus. The action myoclonus may be
responsive to anticonvulsants such as clonazepam or valproate. Experimental use of
5-hydroxytryptophan, a precursor of serotonin, has also been effective.

Case

A 68-year-old woman was brought to the emergency unit pulseless following a
cardiac arrest. Return of spontaneous circulation occurred after 5 min of cardiac
arrest. Sixteen hours after admission, while the patient remained comatose, she
developed generalized myoclonic jerks.

R. Bhidayasiri, D. Tarsy, *Movement Disorders: A Video Atlas*, Current Clinical Neurology,
DOI 10.1007/978-1-60327-426-5_86, © Springer Science+Business Media New York 2012

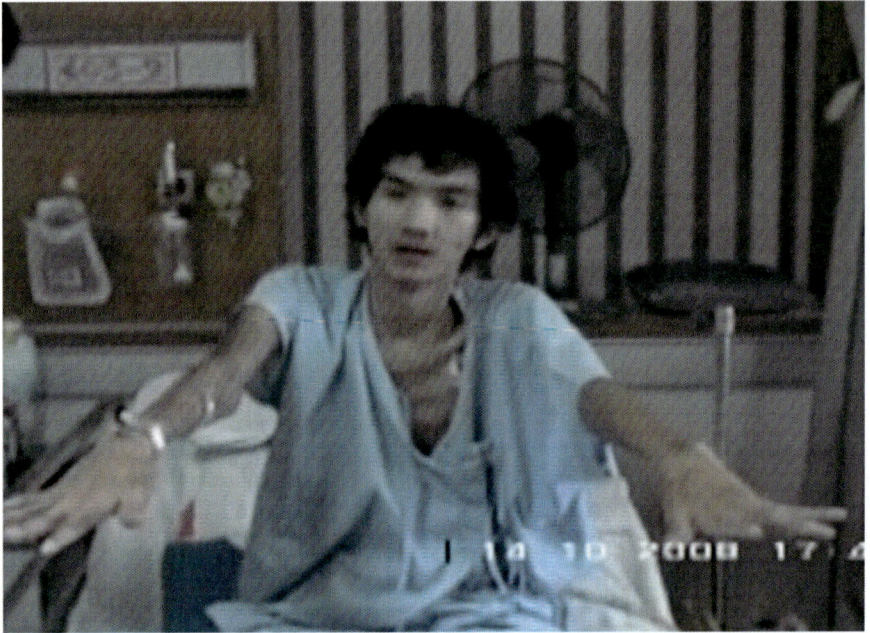

Video

Clip 1: the patient exhibits generalized myoclonic jerks involving her limbs. *Clip 2*: another patient with Lance-Adams Syndrome is seen here 2 years after a respiratory arrest following an asthmatic attack. He shows residual action myoclonus involving both upper limbs. Positive and negative myoclonus are both present. Myoclonic action tremor is evident during finger-chin testing.

References

1. Lance JW, Adams RD. The syndrome of intention or action myoclonus as a sequel to hypoxic encephalopathy. Brain. 1963;86:111–36.
2. Frucht S, Fahn S. The clinical spectrum of posthypoxic myoclonus. Mov Disord. 2000;15 Suppl 1:2–7.
3. Werhahn KJ, Brown P, Thompson PD. The clinical features and prognosis of chronic posthypoxic myoclonus. Mov Disord. 1997;12:216–20.

Chapter 87
Essential Myoclonus

This chapter contains a video segment which can be found at the
URL: http://www.springerimages.com/Tarsy

Background

Myoclonus is either the only or the most prominent finding in essential myoclonus.
Myoclonus is therefore a nearly isolated phenomenon from which the patient usually
experiences relatively mild disability. Essential myoclonus may be sporadic or genetically determined and either does not progress or progresses very slowly over many
years. Hereditary essential myoclonus is characterized by onset before age 20, dominant inheritance with variable severity, a benign clinical course compatible with an
active life and normal longevity, and the absence of other neurological signs. The
myoclonus typically is generalized, is exacerbated by muscle activation, and is sub-
stantially decreased by alcohol ingestion. The term "myoclonus-dystonia" syndrome
has been introduced because of the common occurrence of dystonia in these cases.

Case

A 72-year-old woman was referred because of intermittent generalized twitching.
The patient stated that onset was more than 50 years ago previously. One sibling
was similarly affected. The twitching did not interfere with daily activities, and she
noticed a partial response to alcohol. Examination revealed generalized myoclonus
involving the trunk and all four extremities. Dystonia was absent. The remainder of
the examination was normal.

References

1. Bressman S, Fahn S. Essential myoclonus. Adv Neurol. 1986;43:287–94.
2. Caviness JN, Brown P. Myoclonus: current concepts and recent advances. Lancet Neurol.
   2004;3:598–607.

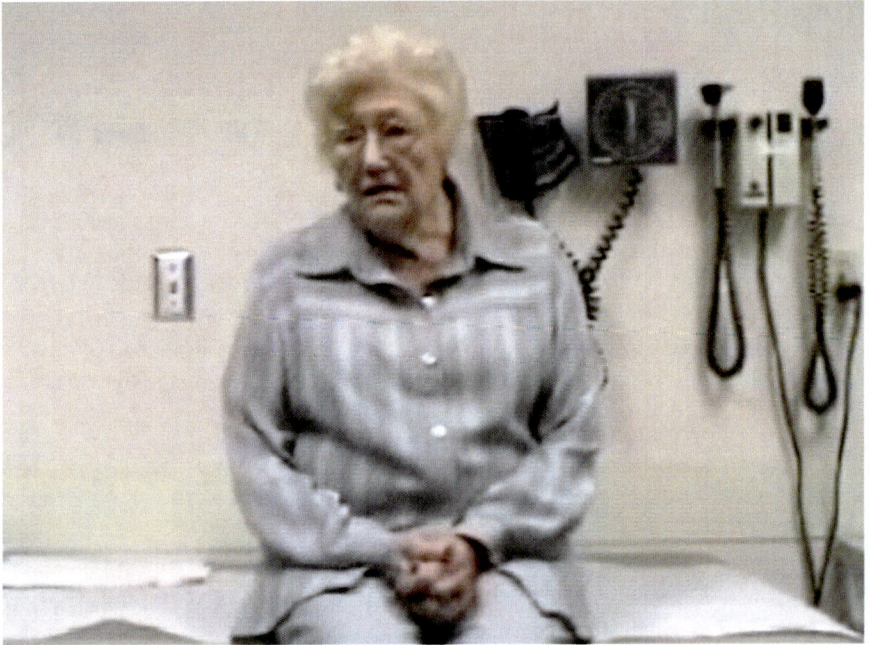

Video
The patient exhibits generalized myoclonus at rest involving the trunk and lower more than upper extremities.

Chapter 88
Negative Myoclonus

This chapter contains a video segment which can be found at the
URL: http://www.springerimages.com/Tarsy

Background

Negative myoclonus refers to an abrupt involuntary movement caused by sudden,
brief interruptions of muscle activity. Recently, the Task Force on Classification and
Terminology of the International League against Epilepsy recognized negative
myoclonus as a seizure type, defining it as an "interruption of tonic muscle activity
for less than 500 ms without evidence of preceding myoclonia." Clinically, negative
myoclonus is classified into four types: asterixis, postural lapses, epileptic negative
myoclonus, and physiologic negative myoclonus. Asterixis, which usually occurs in
metabolic or toxic encephalopathies, is considered to be subcortical in origin but the
cerebral cortex may be involved in some cases. Asterixis also rarely occurs unilaterally following thalamic infarcts. When negative myoclonus involves axial or leg
muscles, patients may fall abruptly resulting in a drop attack. Epileptic negative
myoclonus is defined as an interruption of tonic muscle activity which is time-
locked to an epileptic EEG abnormality without evidence of antecedent positive
myoclonus in agonist or antagonist muscles. Physiologic negative myoclonus occurs
in normal individuals when falling asleep, after prolonged exercise, or when overly
anxious but has not been characterized neurophysiologically.

The clinical features of negative myoclonus may sometimes make it difficult to
distinguish it from positive myoclonus, and in some situations both disorders may
coexist. Therefore, polygraphic monitoring is essential for the diagnosis of negative
myoclonus, allowing for the demonstration of brief interruptions of tonic EMG
activity, not preceded by a positive myoclonic jerk in the agonist and antagonist
muscles of the affected limb.

Case

A 72-year-old man with a history of cryptogenic liver disease was admitted to the
hospital with upper gastrointestinal hemorrhage from esophageal varices. He was
disoriented to time and place. Examination showed sudden involuntary jerky movements of his hands at the wrists which became worse when the patient held his arms
outstretched with his wrists extended.

R. Bhidayasiri, D. Tarsy, *Movement Disorders: A Video Atlas*, Current Clinical Neurology,   190
DOI 10.1007/978-1-60327-426-5_88, © Springer Science+Business Media New York 2012

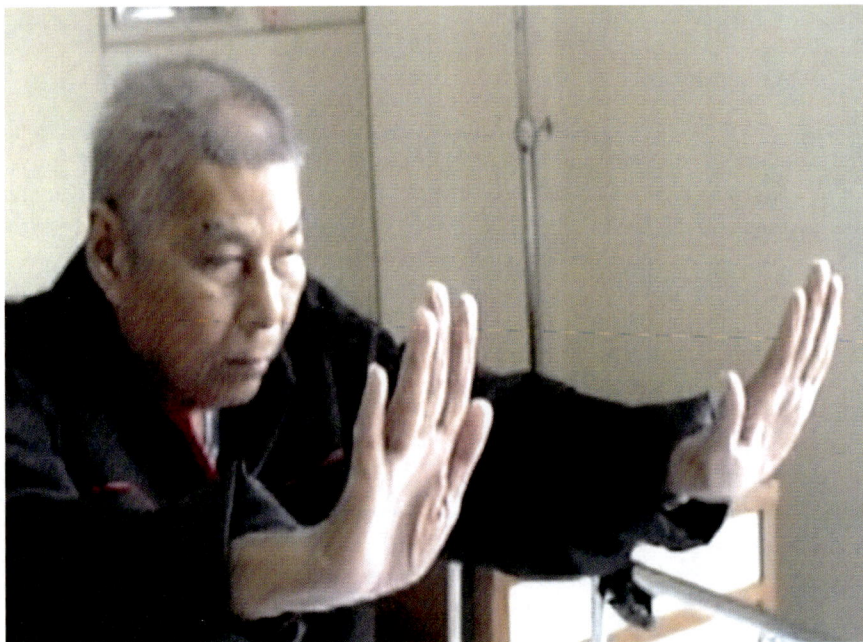

Video

Examination shows an irregular distal upper extremity tremor and sudden jerks involving the hands and fingers bilaterally. When he maintains his hands in an extended posture, the jerky involuntary movements worsen and resemble a flapping tremor. There is an action tremor during finger-nose testing.

References

1. Shibasaki H. Physiology of negative myoclonus. Adv Neurol. 2002;89:103–13.
2. Obeso JA, Artieda J, Burleigh A. Clinical aspects of negative myoclonus. Adv Neurol. 1995;67:1–7.
3. Young RR, Shahani BT. Asterixis, one type of negative myoclonus. Adv Neurol. 1986; 43:137–56.

Chapter 89
Propriospinal Myoclonus

This chapter contains a video segment which can be found at the
URL: http://www.springerimages.com/Tarsy

Background

Propriospinal myoclonus (PSM) is a rare movement disorder characterized by myoclonic jerks in muscles believed to originate in a myoclonic generator (a "myelom-
ere") which spread rostrally and caudally to other myotomes above and below the
generator. Characteristic features include repetitive, arrhythmic flexion jerks of the
trunk, hips, and knees. The signal spreads slowly along propriospinal pathways.
Propriospinal myoclonus is idiopathic and has occurred following spinal cord
lesions, spinal trauma, drug use, tumor, or infections. However, a specific cause is
identified in only 20% of patients. Most affected patients are middle-aged men. In
most cases, the myoclonic generator is at the thoracic level. Diagnosis is based on
the characteristic clinical features mentioned above and polymyography which
shows a slow and orderly rostrocaudal propagation of muscle recruitment.
Conventional spinal cord MRI is typically normal. Psychogenic myoclonus may
present with features of PSM, and a recording of cortical activity immediately preceding the jerks is recommended as a control since the premovement potential
(Bereitschaftspotential) is present only immediately before voluntary movements.

Symptomatic therapy is often disappointing, and there are no guidelines for therapy selections. The most commonly effective treatment is clonazepam or other benzodiazepines which result in only mild to moderate improvement. Valproate and
zonisamide have also been reported to be helpful.

Case

Following drug intoxication, a 45-year-old woman developed involuntary generalized body myoclonus causing sudden flexion jerks at the hips, neck, and trunk. The
frequency and severity of the jerks increased while lying supine, but the jerks were
also present while sitting or standing. Myoclonus was provoked by cutaneous stimuli to the chest, abdomen, and back. Tendon reflexes were brisk with extensor plantar responses, but the rest of the neurological examination was normal. Brain and
complete spinal cord MRI were normal.

R. Bhidayasiri, D. Tarsy, *Movement Disorders: A Video Atlas*, Current Clinical Neurology,
DOI 10.1007/978-1-60327-426-5_89, © Springer Science+Business Media New York 2012

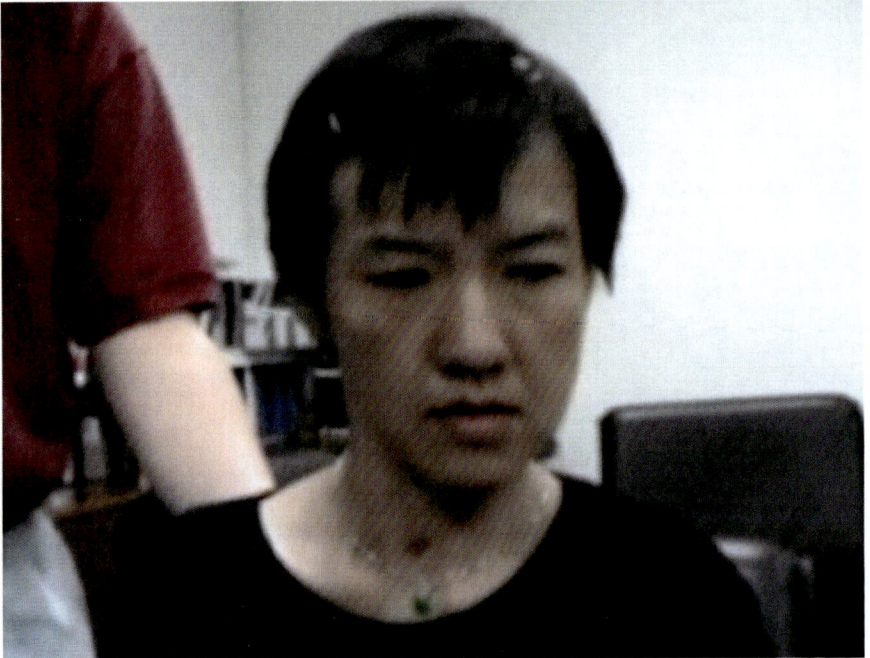

Video
The video demonstrates that cutaneous stimuli to the back, chest, and abdomen elicit axial myo-clonic jerks which cause low-amplitude flexion movements of the hips, neck, trunk, and right sternomastoid muscle while the patient is standing. There is mild scoliosis.

References

1. Brown P, Thompson PD, Rothwell JC. Axial myoclonus of propriospinal origin. Brain. 1991;114:197–214.
2. Roze E, Bounolleau P, Ducreux D, et al. Propriospinal myoclonus revisited. Clinical, neuro-physiologic, and neuroradiologic findings. Neurology. 2009;72:1301–9.

Chapter 90
Myoclonus-Dystonia Syndrome

This chapter contains a video segment which can be found at the
URL: http://www.springerimages.com/Tarsy

Background

Myoclonus-dystonia (M-D) is a genetically heterogeneous movement disorder with
autosomal dominant inheritance. Clinically, the disorder is characterized by myoclonic jerks and dystonic movements which characteristically respond to alcohol.
Psychiatric abnormalities are often a part of the phenotype. A major gene locus
maps to the epsilon-sarcoglycan gene (SGCE, DYT11) on chromosome 7q21-22,
which encodes a transmembrane protein that is widely expressed in the brain but is
of unknown function. A classification of M-D diagnostic categories was recently
proposed: Definite M-D refers to early onset myoclonus and dystonia or isolated
myoclonus occurring predominantly in the upper half of the body with a positive
family history for myoclonus and/or dystonia. Probable M-D is the same but without a family history. Possible M-D refers to jerky dystonia of the neck or isolated
jerky movements of variable distribution or with signs of dystonia and/or myoclonus in the lower body half and no response to alcohol.

Since patients with essential myoclonus sometimes also display dystonia (see
Chap. 87), it is increasingly recognized that the relation between essential myoclonus and M-D is complex. Indeed, many experts suggest that hereditary essential
myoclonus and dominantly inherited M-D with lightning jerks and dramatic
response to alcohol may be the same disorder.

Case

A 22-year-old man presented with intermittent jerky movements of both hands
which had progressively become more pronounced so as to interfere with his work
as a mechanic. He was initially diagnosed with epilepsy, but this diagnosis was challenged by his primary physician and he was referred. Examination revealed myoclonic jerks which predominantly involved his upper limbs and neck. He also had
dynamic retrocollis with superimposed jerky head movements. The jerks responded
dramatically to alcohol.

R. Bhidayasiri, D. Tarsy, *Movement Disorders: A Video Atlas*, Current Clinical Neurology,
DOI 10.1007/978-1-60327-426-5_90, © Springer Science+Business Media New York 2012

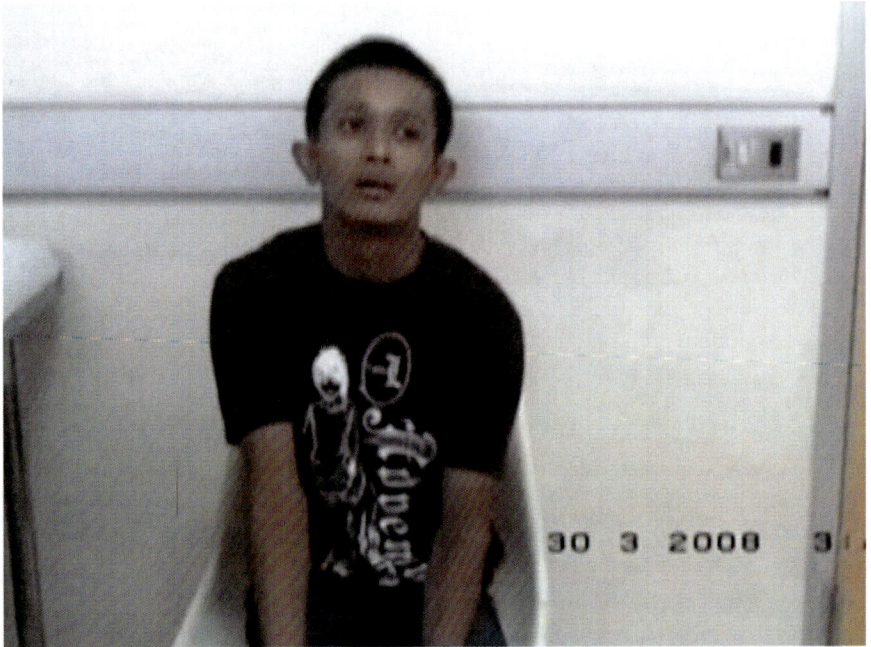

Video

The patient exhibits myoclonic jerks which predominantly involve his hands and fingers bilaterally, occurring both at rest and during action. Axial jerks are occasionally present. In addition, dynamic retrocollis is prominent with superimposed myoclonic jerks of the head. Mild blepharospasm is also present.

References

1. Quinn NP. Essential myoclonus and myoclonic dystonia. Mov Disord. 1996;11:119–24.
2. Grunewald A, Djarmati A, Lohmann-Hedrich K, et al. Myoclonus-dystonia: significance of large SGCE deletions. Hum Mutat. 2008;29:331–2.
3. Ritz K, Gerrits MCF, Foncke EMJ, et al. Myoclonus-dystonia: clinical and genetic evaluation of a large cohort. J Neurol Neurosurg Psychiatry. 2009;80:653–8.

Chapter 91
Opsoclonus-Myoclonus-Ataxia Syndrome

This chapter contains a video segment which can be found at the
URL: http://www.springerimages.com/Tarsy

Background

Opsoclonus-myoclonus-ataxia syndrome (OMA) typically causes opsoclonus (con-
jugate, multidirectional chaotic eye movements), myoclonus, and ataxia, sometimes
together with sleep disorders, cognitive deficit, and behavioral disturbance.
Myoclonus is brief and spontaneous, usually with stimulus-sensitive jerks involving
the limbs, palate, face, larynx, or respiratory muscles. The syndrome can develop
subacutely or progress quickly.

   Causes of OMA may be categorized by age of onset. In children, OMA occurs
most frequently in females between 6 months and 3 years. OMA is sometimes paraneoplastic and should be suspected where it is not preceded by a definite infection.
Neuroblastoma is found in more than 50% of cases. Symptoms and signs may remit
spontaneously but relapses are common. After exclusion of structural or infectious
causes, OMA may prove to be either paraneoplastic or idiopathic. In adults, in most
cases OMA precedes the diagnosis of tumor. Median age of onset is 66 in paraneoplastic cases and 40 in idiopathic cases. Encephalopathy is almost exclusively seen
in the paraneoplastic group which is usually related to small cell lung cancer or
breast cancer. In most cases, CSF and brain MRI are unremarkable or reveal
nonspecific changes in brainstem and cerebellum. Antibody tests are usually negative, but some studies have reported IgM and IgG antibodies that bind to Purkinje
cell cytoplasm. Spontaneous resolution or response to immunotherapy occasionally
occurs, especially among idiopathic cases. Survival in adults with paraneoplastic
OMA is related to the responsiveness of the underlying tumor and its prognosis.

Case

A previously healthy 25-year-old man developed sudden gait unsteadiness and body
jerks following a 2-week history of low-grade fever and malaise. During the subsequent week, symptoms gradually worsened to include unsteadiness, tremors, vomiting, vertigo, and diplopia. Examination revealed opsoclonus and coarse bilateral hand
tremor. He became bed-bound with marked truncal ataxia and myoclonic jerks of the
face, head, trunk, and extremities to the extent that he could not sit up in bed. CBC,
chemistries, chest X-ray, and brain MRI were normal. Extensive investigations did not
reveal any tumor but he was HIV-seropositive. After 3 weeks of supportive therapy,
his condition gradually improved with nearly complete recovery at 3 months.

R. Bhidayasiri, D. Tarsy, *Movement Disorders: A Video Atlas*, Current Clinical Neurology,   196
DOI 10.1007/978-1-60327-426-5_91, © Springer Science+Business Media New York 2012

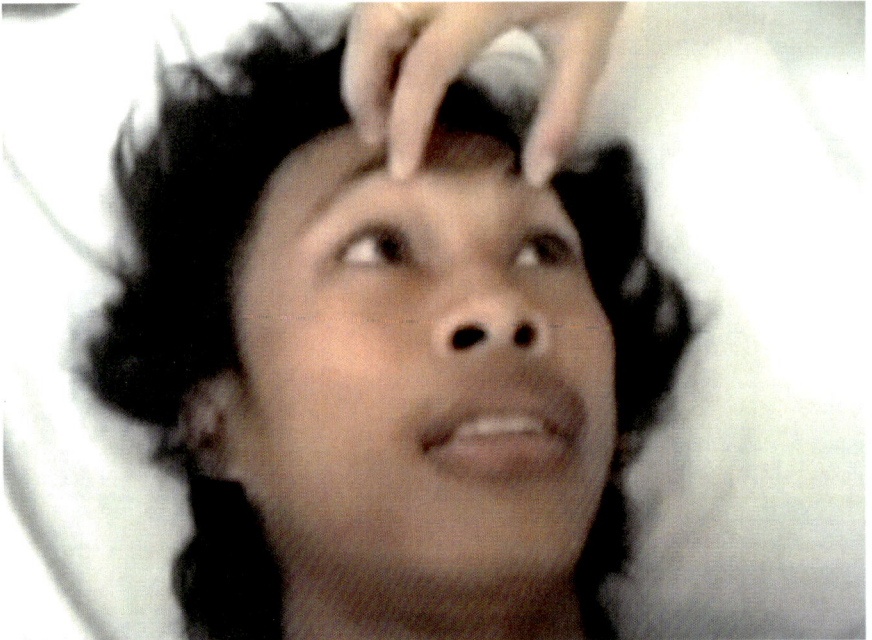

Video
Clip 1: The patient exhibits severe, high-frequency generalized myoclonic jerks and opsoclonus.
Clip 2: Examination 3 months after onset shows almost complete recovery except for mild bilateral action tremor.

References

1. Pang KK, de Sousa C, Lang B. A prospective study of the presentation and management of dancing eye syndrome/opsoclonus-myoclonus syndrome in the United Kingdom. Eur J Paediatr Neurol. 2010;14:156–61.
2. Bataller L, Graus F, Saiz A, et al. Clinical outcome in adult onset idiopathic or paraneoplastic opsoclonus-myoclonus. Brain. 2001;124:437–43.
3. Kanjanasut N, Phanthumchinda K, Bhidayasiri R. HIV-related opsoclonus-myoclonus-ataxia syndrome: report on two cases. Clin Neurol Neurosurg. 2010;112:572–4.

Chapter 92
Progressive Myoclonic Epilepsy

This chapter contains a video segment which can be found at the
URL: http://www.springerimages.com/Tarsy

Background

Myoclonic seizures are epileptic seizures in which the main manifestation is myoclonus. Myoclonus is accompanied by a generalized epileptiform discharge but the
myoclonus may be generalized, segmental, or focal. Progressive myoclonic epilepsies (PMEs) are an unusual and heterogeneous group of epilepsies with debilitating
progression, resistance to conventional treatment, and poor prognosis. Although
initial manifestations may be similar to idiopathic generalized epilepsies or juvenile
myoclonic epilepsy, therapeutic failure and progressive worsening of neurological
signs suggest PME. Despite its broad clinical spectrum, PME has several distinctive
clinical characteristics including myoclonus, multiple seizure types, delay or regres-
sion in psychomotor development, and cerebellar signs. PME usually begins in
childhood and adolescence and constitutes approximately 1% of epileptic syndromes in these age groups. In PME, myoclonus is typically precipitated by postural changes, action, or external sensory stimuli to the face and distal extremities.

PME includes a number of separate disorders, including Unverricht-Lundborg
disease, myoclonic epilepsy with ragged red fibers, neuronal ceroid lipofuscinosis,
dentatorubral-pallidoluysian atrophy, and Lafora's disease. The example presented
here is Lafora's disease which is an autosomal recessive disorder characterized by
epilepsy, myoclonus, dementia, and pathognomonic inclusion bodies of Lafora
found within neurons, cardiac cells, skeletal muscle, liver, and sebaceous gland
ducts. Mutations in EPM2A/laforin are the cause of 58% of cases, while mutations
in EPM2B/malin are the cause of 35% of cases.

Case

The patient is a 25-year-old woman who experienced the onset of seizures at age 19.
Her seizures were of multiple types and included episodes of status epilepticus. In
addition to myoclonic seizures, cognitive function had deteriorated and there was
ataxia, dysarthria, and visual impairment. Her myoclonus was of several types
including spontaneous, action, multifocal, and generalized. The diagnosis of
Lafora's disease was confirmed by a skin biopsy showing inclusion bodies of Lafora,
which are periodic-acid-Schiff positive polyglucosans.

R. Bhidayasiri, D. Tarsy, *Movement Disorders: A Video Atlas*, Current Clinical Neurology,   198
DOI 10.1007/978-1-60327-426-5_92, © Springer Science+Business Media New York 2012

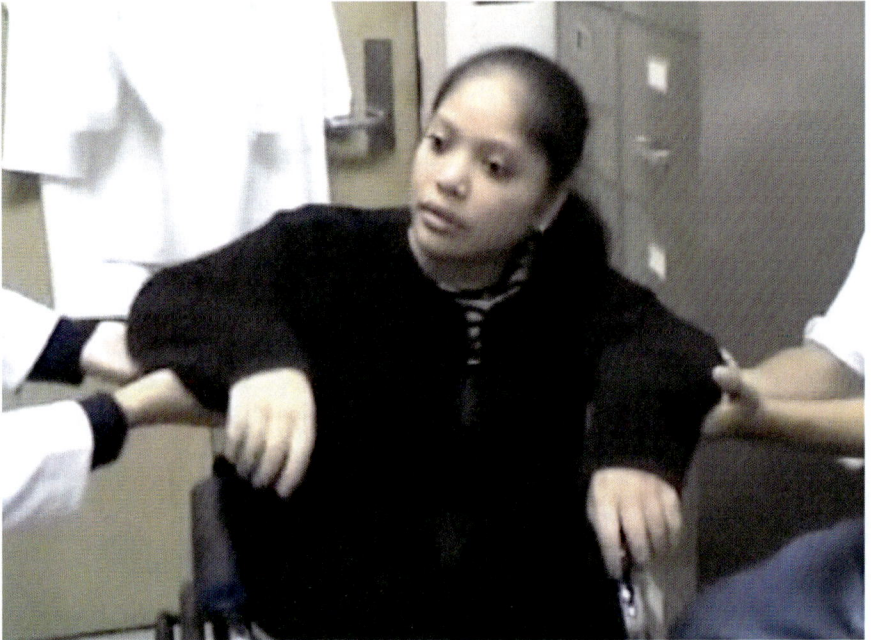

Video
The patient exhibits multifocal action myoclonus involving the face, trunk, and extremities. (Video contribution from Dr. AV. Delgado-Escueta, UCLA.)

References

1. Shahwan A, Farrell M, Delanty N. Progressive myoclonic epilepsies: a review of genetic and therapeutic aspects. Lancet Neurol. 2005;4:239–48.
2. Delgado-Escueta AV. Advances in Lafora progressive myoclonus epilepsy. Curr Neurol Neurosci Rep. 2007;7:428–33.

Chapter 93
Hemifacial Spasm

This chapter contains a video segment which can be found at the
URL: http://www.springerimages.com/Tarsy

Background

Hemifacial spasm (HFS) is a form of peripheral myoclonus, characterized by progressive, involuntary, irregular, and clonic or sometimes more long-lasting tonic
movements of muscles innervated by the seventh cranial nerve on one side of the
face. The upper and/or lower eyelids are the most common site of initial involvement, followed by the cheek and perioral regions. Complete unilateral eye closure
may interfere with vision and cause social embarrassment. HFS is relatively uncommon but is a disturbing symptom when it occurs. Mean age of onset is 49 years, and
there is a slight female preponderance. The most frequent cause of HFS is compression of the facial nerve at the pontine root exit zone by an ectopic anatomical or
pathological structure which results in ephaptic transmission. The anterior or posterior inferior cerebellar and vertebral arteries or their branches are most commonly
involved, but compression by an atherosclerotic, aberrant, and ectatic basilar artery
may also cause HFS which in rare cases may be bilateral. Coronal MRI with thin
cuts through the posterior fossa usually reveals any existing compressive lesion.
Facial nerve injury or a prior Bell's palsy may also cause HFS which is usually more
tonic, usually unassociated with clonic facial movements, and is often accompanied
by synkinetic "crocodile tears" while eating. Botulinum toxin provides moderate to
marked improvement in 95% of patients and is considered the treatment of choice.
Anticonvulsant medications are commonly used but are rarely effective.
Microvascular decompression (MD) was formally used to treat HFS but currently is
limited to severe cases in which botulinum toxin is or has become ineffective.
Although MD is successful in 90% of cases, HFS may recur within a year or occasionally is associated with transient or permanent surgical complications such as
ipsilateral hearing loss or facial weakness.

Case

A 45-year-old woman was experiencing right facial twitching for 2 years. The
spasms had gradually worsened and began to interfere with vision. Examination
revealed right HFS confined to muscles innervated by the right facial nerve. There
was no evidence of hearing loss, facial numbness, facial pain, or other cranial nerve
abnormalities. Brain MRI showed vascular indentation in the right pons at the root
exit zone of the right facial nerve.

R. Bhidayasiri, D. Tarsy, *Movement Disorders: A Video Atlas*, Current Clinical Neurology,
DOI 10.1007/978-1-60327-426-5_93, © Springer Science+Business Media New York 2012

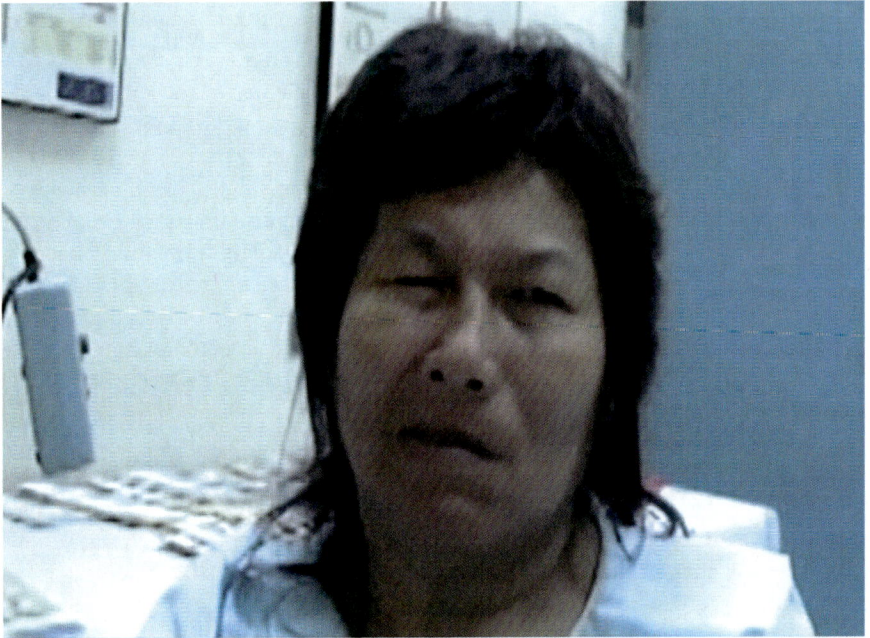

Video
The patient exhibits continuous tonic right HFS involving predominantly orbicularis oculi, zygomaticus major, nasalis, and platysma muscles.

References

1. Wang A, Jankovic J. Hemifacial spasm: clinical findings and treatment. Muscle Nerve. 1998;21:1740–7.
2. Adler CA, Zimmerman RA, Savino PJ, et al. Hemifacial spasm: evaluation by magnetic resonance imaging and magnetic resonance tomographic angiography. Ann Neurol. 1992;32:502–6.
3. Jitpimolmard S, Tiamkao S, Laopaiboon M. Long term results of botulinum toxin type A (Dysport) in the treatment of hemifacial spasm: a report of 175 cases. J Neurol Neurosurg Psychiatry. 1998;64:751–7.

Chapter 94
Epilepsia Partialis Continua

This chapter contains a video segment which can be found at the
URL: http://www.springerimages.com/Tarsy

Background

Epilepsia partialis continua (EPC) is a rare form of focal status epilepticus characterized by continuous regular or irregular clonic muscular twitching affecting a limited part of the body, sometimes aggravated by action or sensory stimuli, and
occurring for a minimum of 1 h. Neurophysiologically, the diagnosis of EPC
requires the demonstration of epileptiform EEG abnormalities, ideally with a fixed
temporal association with the muscle jerks. Other abnormalities may include giant
somatosensory-evoked potentials which demonstrate the cortical origin of the muscle jerks. EPC has been linked with both motor cortex and adjacent subcortical
discharges. EPC may be due to vascular lesions (14%), inflammatory disorders
(32%), head trauma (16%), neoplastic disorders (19%), and unknown causes (16%).
Rasmussen's encephalitis is the most common cause of EPC in childhood.

A common clinical sign of EPC is the combination of muscle jerks together with
hemiparesis causing simple, brief excursions of the affected limb. The jerks can be
regular or irregular with more involvement of distal than proximal muscle groups.
Physical exercise and psychic stimulation may increase the amplitude and frequency
of the jerks. EPC may mimic focal myoclonus or tremor. The upper limbs are
affected three times more commonly than the lower limbs.

Case

A 38-year-old man presented with repetitive jerks of the right arm following an
episode of right-sided weakness. Examination showed regular muscle jerks involving the right arm which were more prominent distally than proximally. Individual
episodes lasted for hours at a time. The patient was aware of the jerks and was fully
alert throughout the episode.

References

1. Engel Jr J. A proposed diagnostic scheme for people with epileptic seizures and with epilepsy:
   report of the ILAE Task Force on classification and terminology. Epilepsia. 2001;42:796–803.
2. Cockerell OC, Rothwell J, Thompson PD, et al. Clinical and physiological features of epilepsia
   partialise continua. Cases ascertained in the UK. Brain. 1996;119:393–407.
3. Bien CG, Elger CE. Epilepsia partialis continua: semiology and differential diagnoses. Epileptic
   Disord. 2008;10:3–7.

R. Bhidayasiri, D. Tarsy, *Movement Disorders: A Video Atlas*, Current Clinical Neurology,   202
DOI 10.1007/978-1-60327-426-5_94, © Springer Science+Business Media New York 2012

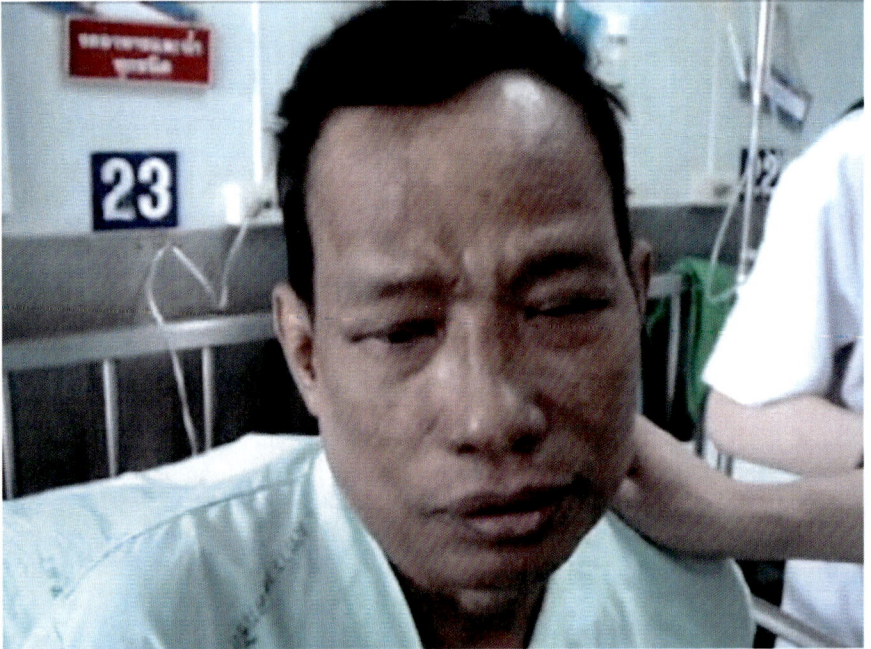

Video
The patient exhibits a train of regular jerks involving the right upper limb which are more prominent in the arm and elbow (Video contribution from Dr. Helen Ling, Chiang Mai University Hospital, Thailand).

Chapter 95
Anti-NMDA-Receptor Encephalitis

This chapter contains a video segment which can be found at the
URL: http://www.springerimages.com/Tarsy

Background

N-methyl-D-aspartate (NMDA) receptors are ligand-gated cation channels with cru-
cial roles in synaptic transmission and plasticity. Anti-NMDA-receptor encephalitis
is associated with antibodies against NR1-NR2 heteromers and is characterized by
a combination of neuropsychiatric symptoms, seizures, alteration of consciousness,
movement disorders, and autonomic instability. Most patients are women with a
median age of 23 years. Sixty percent of patients have tumors, most commonly
ovarian teratomas, but the absence of an identifiable tumor is common. The movement disorders associated with this syndrome consist of semirhythmic repetitive
bulbar and limb movements which persist during prolonged periods of unrespon-
siveness. The mechanism underlying the abnormal movements is believed to be an
interruption of forebrain corticostriatal inputs by anti-NMDA receptor antibodies
that remove tonic inhibition of brainstem pattern generators which in turn releases
primitive patterns of bulbar and limb movements. Patients who undergo early tumor
removal together with immunotherapy have better outcomes with fewer neurological relapses. Improvement is associated with a decrease in NMDA antibody levels.
Early recognition and treatment of this disorder leads to better outcomes.

Case

A 21-year-old woman presented after 2 weeks of mental confusion, agitation, headaches, and increasing somnolence. Examination revealed rhythmic chewing movements and lip pouting. There was frequent facial grimacing with elevations of the
eyes. Oral movements appeared to be synchronized with complex movements in the
upper and lower limbs, which consisted mainly of repetitive finger flexion and hip
flexion movements with internal rotation of the legs. There were intermittent ballistic movements of the arms. All movements were refractory to sedating drugs. The
patient had fluctuating periods of altered awareness, partly due to generalized tonic-
clonic seizures. Anti-NMDA-receptor antibodies were detected by Prof. Angela
Vincent (University of Oxford). Extensive investigations did not identify an underlying tumor.

R. Bhidayasiri, D. Tarsy, *Movement Disorders: A Video Atlas*, Current Clinical Neurology,   204
DOI 10.1007/978-1-60327-426-5_95, © Springer Science+Business Media New York 2012

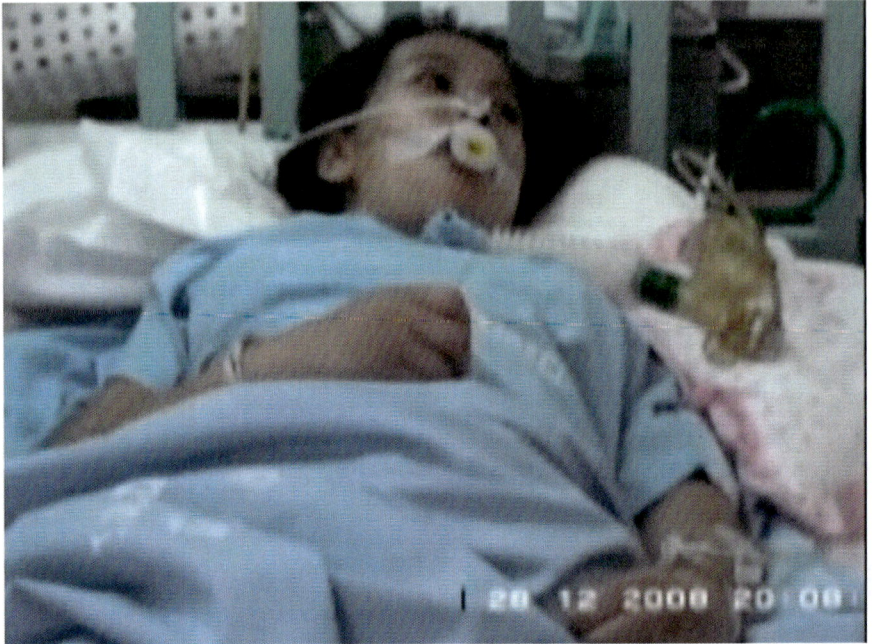

Video
The patient exhibits complex involuntary movements consisting of rhythmic chewing movements and facial grimacing together with stereotypic jerking movements of the hands and legs.

References

1. Kleinig TJ, Thompson PD, Matar W, et al. The distinctive movement disorder of ovarian teratoma-associated encephalitis. Mov Disord. 2008;23:1256–61.
2. Dalmau J, Tuzun E, Wu HY, et al. Paraneoplastic anti-N-methyl-D-aspartate receptor encephalitis associated with ovarian teratoma. Ann Neurol. 2007;61:25–36.
3. Dalmau J, Gleichman A, Hughes EG, et al. Anti-NMDA-receptor encephalitis: case series and analysis of the effects of antibodies. Lancet Neurol. 2008;7:1091–8.

Chapter 96
Psychogenic Myoclonus

This chapter contains a video segment which can be found at the
URL: http://www.springerimages.com/Tarsy

Background

Generalized and focal stimulus-sensitive muscle jerks often represent a form of abnormal startle response or reflex myoclonus. However, these movements may also occur
as a psychogenic movement disorder. Indeed, psychogenic myoclonus or muscle jerks
represent a common form of psychogenic movement disorder, accounting for 8.5% of
patients with myoclonus and 20% of psychogenic movement disorders. Distinguishing
between psychogenic myoclonus and other forms of myoclonus may be difficult. A
number of characteristic features of psychogenic myoclonus/jerks have been proposed
including (1) the inconsistent character of the movements which are incongruous with
typical organic myoclonus, (2) obvious reduction of myoclonus with distraction, (3)
exacerbation and relief with placebo and suggestion, (4) spontaneous periods of
remission, (5) acute onset and sudden resolution, and (6) evidence for underlying
psychopathology. Neurophysiologic observations indicate that movements of psychogenic origin are characterized by variable latencies to onset of stimulus-induced jerks,
longer latencies than those which occur in reflex myoclonus, variable patterns of muscle recruitment within each jerk, and habituation with repeated stimulation.

Case

A previously healthy 35-year-old woman acutely developed generalized body jerks
unaccompanied by seizures or loss of consciousness. Examination showed absence
of myoclonus at rest or while active. However, a sudden sound, such as a loud clap,
produced a generalized whole body "jump," sometimes followed by a series of small
"jumps" with variable amplitude. She remained alert and was able to communicate
throughout the examination. Loud sounds while she was walking produced a similar
reaction but did not cause her to fall. The movements subsided when she was treated
with an antidepressant and recurred when the medication was withdrawn.

References

1. Thompson PD, Colebatch JG, Brown P, et al. Voluntary stimulus-sensitive jerks and jumps
   mimicking myoclonus or pathological startle syndromes. Mov Disord. 1992;7:257–62.
2. Monday K, Jankovic J. Psychogenic myoclonus. Neurology. 1993;43:349–52.

R. Bhidayasiri, D. Tarsy, *Movement Disorders: A Video Atlas*, Current Clinical Neurology,
DOI 10.1007/978-1-60327-426-5_96, © Springer Science+Business Media New York 2012

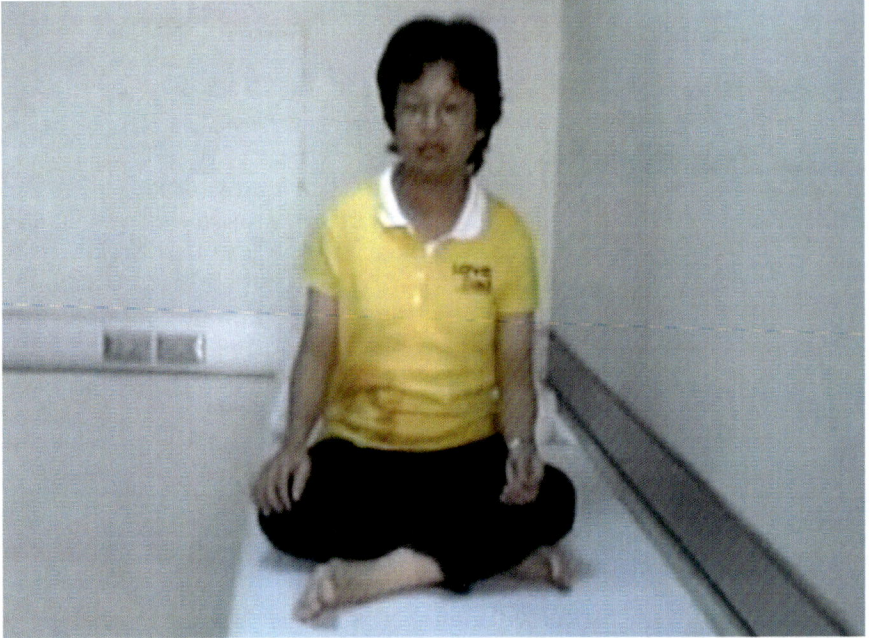

Video
While supine, the patient exhibits a generalized body jerk characterized by hip and variable elbow flexion following loud claps. While sitting, with a more prolonged latency following a loud clap, she develops a sudden whole body jerk with milder hip flexion and bilateral arm flexion to head level.

Part VI
Cerebellar Ataxia

Chapter 97
Cerebellar Ataxia Type 1

This chapter contains a video segment which can be found at the
URL: http://www.springerimages.com/Tarsy

Background

Spinocerebellar ataxia-type 1 (SCA1) was the first dominantly inherited ataxia for
which the locus and gene defect were identified. SCA1 is caused by polyQ-encoding CAG repeat expansions resulting in production of the abnormal protein,
Ataxin-1. Similar to other polyQ diseases, SCA1 shows considerable phenotypic
variability and anticipation that reflects differences in repeat size among affected
individuals. Most patients present in the fourth decade with a pancerebellar syndrome including ataxia of gait, stance, and limbs and dysarthria. Oculomotor abnormalities include gaze-evoked nystagmus, saccadic hypermetria, breakdown of
smooth pursuit eye movements, and reduced opticokinetic nystagmus. In most
patients, there are additional noncerebellar signs. Spasticity with extensor plantar
responses and hyperreflexia occur in more than 50% of SCA1 patients. Reduced
vibration sense is present in 80% of patients, and dysphagia is an important clinical
problem in late stages of the disease. Chorea, stridor, and vocal cord paralysis sometimes develop as the disease advances. Executive dysfunction is common but rarely
progresses to frank dementia. Nevertheless, the above-mentioned physical signs
may not differentiate SCA1 from other SCA subtypes. Although SCA1 is not the
most common form of SCA, it is better understood at the molecular level than other
SCAs, and studies of this disease continue to lead the way in our understanding of
the entire class of polyQ neurodegenerative disorders.

Case

A 57-year-old man was referred for staggering gait and inability to walk straight
together with slurred speech. Symptoms began at age 45 and slowly progressed.
Several ancestors were reported to have gait problems but details were not available.
Examination revealed dysarthric speech, a wide-based gait, and poor tandem gait.
Hyperreflexia was present in both legs but plantar responses were flexor. Genetic
tests showed an abnormal expansion of CAG repeats on the SCA1 gene.

R. Bhidayasiri, D. Tarsy, *Movement Disorders: A Video Atlas*, Current Clinical Neurology,
DOI 10.1007/978-1-60327-426-5_97, © Springer Science+Business Media New York 2012

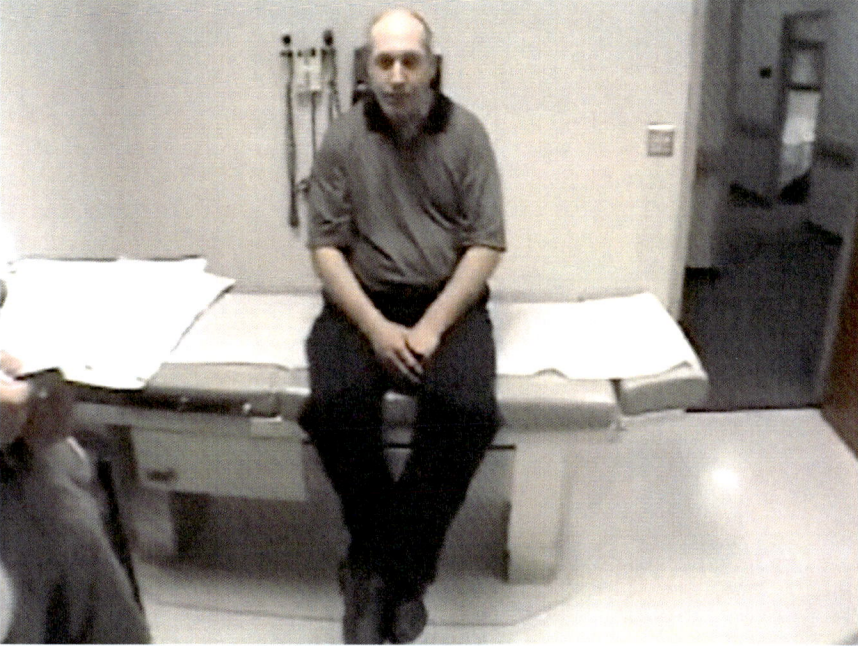

Video
The patient is being examined for cerebellar signs. He is able to walk independently but unsteadily. His gait is slightly wide-based. He performs tandem gait with difficulty with a tendency to veer to the right. Tandem stance and heel-knee-shin testing are normal. Speech is slow and dysarthric with a monotonous low-pitch tone. (Video contribution from Dr. Susan Perlman, Department of Neurology at David Geffen School of Medicine at UCLA.)

References

1. Zoghbi HY, Orr HT. Pathogenic mechanisms of a polyglutamine-mediated neurodegenerative disease, spinocerebellar ataxia type 1. J Biol Chem. 2009;284(12):7425–9.
2. Sasaki H, Fukazawa T, Yanagihara T, et al. Clinical features and natural history of spinocerebellar ataxia type 1. Acta Neurol Scand. 1996;93:64–71.

Chapter 98
Spinocerebellar Ataxia-Type 2

This chapter contains a video segment which can be found at the
URL: http://www.springerimages.com/Tarsy

Background

Spinocerebellar ataxia-type 2 (SCA2) is an autosomal dominant cerebellar ataxia
which commonly presents with ataxia, slow saccadic eye movements, dysarthria,
and peripheral neuropathy. SCA2 is caused by polyQ-encoding CAG repeat expansions resulting in the production of the abnormal protein, Ataxin-2. Normal alleles
are between 15 and 32 repeats in length, while expanded alleles are 53–77 repeats
in length. SCA2 differs clinically from SCA1 in that saccadic slowing, hyporeflexia,
tremor, and titubation are more pronounced. Among the physical signs observed in
SCA2, saccadic slowing is a very characteristic feature which is observed in most
patients. About 50% of patients have vertical or horizontal gaze palsy. Other cerebellar oculomotor abnormalities occur only rarely in SCA2. By contrast with SCA1,
pyramidal tract signs are present in less than 20% of patients but vibration sense is
reduced in most cases while pinprick sensation is otherwise normal.

Atypical SCA2 phenotypes are recognized including those with prominent
dementia, a motor neuron disease-like presentation, levodopa-responsive parkinsonism, and cervical dystonia. These patients often have shorter expansions than the
more common SCA2 patients with prominent ataxia.

Case

A 52-year-old woman presented with a gradual decline in ambulation over 5 years.
Although she complained that her legs were weak, examination disclosed normal
strength in all extremities. Saccadic eye movements were very slow in all directions,
and her gait was markedly ataxic requiring a walker for support. There was an
abnormal expansion of CAG repeats in the SCA2 gene.

References

1. Schols L, Gispert S, Vorgerd M, et al. Spinocerebellar ataxia type 2-genotype and phenotype in
   German kindreds. Arch Neurol. 1997;54:1073–80.
2. Geschwind DH, Perlman S, Figueroa CP, et al. The prevalence and wide clinical spectrum of
   the spinocerebellar ataxia type 2 trinucleotide repeat in patients with autosomal dominant cerebellar ataxia. Am J Hum Genet. 1997;60(4):842–50.

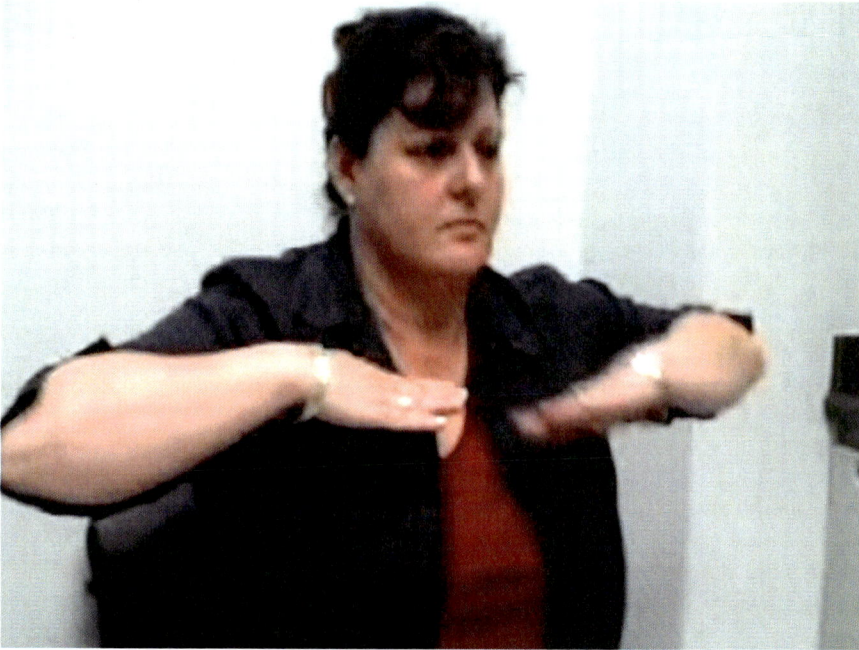

Video

Clip 1: slow saccades are present in both vertical and horizontal directions. Ophthalmoparesis is also evident in all directions. *Clip 2*: examination of another patient with SCA2 reveals mild but definite finger-nose ataxia on the left. Rebound dysmetria is present when she is asked to follow the examiner's fingers with her fingers. *Clip 3*: the patient performs tandem gait with difficulty and has a tendency to veer laterally, more to the right side. (Video contributions from Dr. Susan Perlman, Department of Neurology at David Geffen School of Medicine at UCLA.)

Chapter 99
Spinocerebellar Ataxia-Type 3

This chapter contains a video segment which can be found at the
URL: http://www.springerimages.com/Tarsy

Background

Spinocerebellar ataxia-type 3 (SCA3) or Machado-Joseph disease (MJD) is a clinically heterogeneous, neurodegenerative disorder characterized by varying degrees
of ataxia, ophthalmoplegia, peripheral neuropathy, pyramidal dysfunction, and
movement disorder. It is the most common SCA with a worldwide distribution and,
contrary to early reports, is not limited to individuals of Azorean ancestry. MJD/
SCA3 is caused by CAG repeat expansion mutations in the protein coding region of
the ATXN3 gene located at chromosome 14q32.1. Expanded CAG repeat lengths
correlate with the range and severity of clinical manifestations and inversely correlate with age of disease onset.

Classically, patients with MJD/SCA3 are grouped into five clinically defined
subtypes. However, overlapping features are frequent. Most patients first notice disability due to cerebellar ataxia in their third and fourth decades. Patients often have
diplopia, and the ocular examination reveals gaze-evoked nystagmus, slow saccades
with smooth pursuit eye movements, and supranuclear gaze palsy. A bulging appearance of the eyes is common due to the combination of lid retraction and reduced
blink frequency. Spasticity in the legs is also common, especially in individuals
with early onset disease and large CAG repeat expansions. Two distinctive movement disorders are common, dystonia and parkinsonism. Dystonia usually occurs in
early onset patients and is sometimes task-specific. Parkinsonism is usually bilateral
and symmetrical and often levodopa-responsive. Peripheral neuropathy occurs in
60% of patients, usually in the form of a sensory neuropathy with widespread areas
of tactile and proprioceptive sensory deficit. Recently, restless legs syndrome has
been found to occur in 50% of patients as well as REM sleep behavior disorder,
chronic leg pain, and cramps.

Case

A 42-year-old man was referred with a 2 year history of progressive gait ataxia leading to wheelchair confinement. Speech was dysarthric and hypophonic with frequent dysphagia and regurgitation of food. Examination revealed marked intention
tremor, scanning dysarthria, and a right laterocollis. Ophthalmoplegia, brisk reflexes,
and leg spasticity were also present. His father was similarly affected and processed
a MJD/SCA3 gene mutation with 65 CAG repeats at MJD1.

R. Bhidayasiri, D. Tarsy, *Movement Disorders: A Video Atlas*, Current Clinical Neurology,
DOI 10.1007/978-1-60327-426-5_99, © Springer Science+Business Media New York 2012

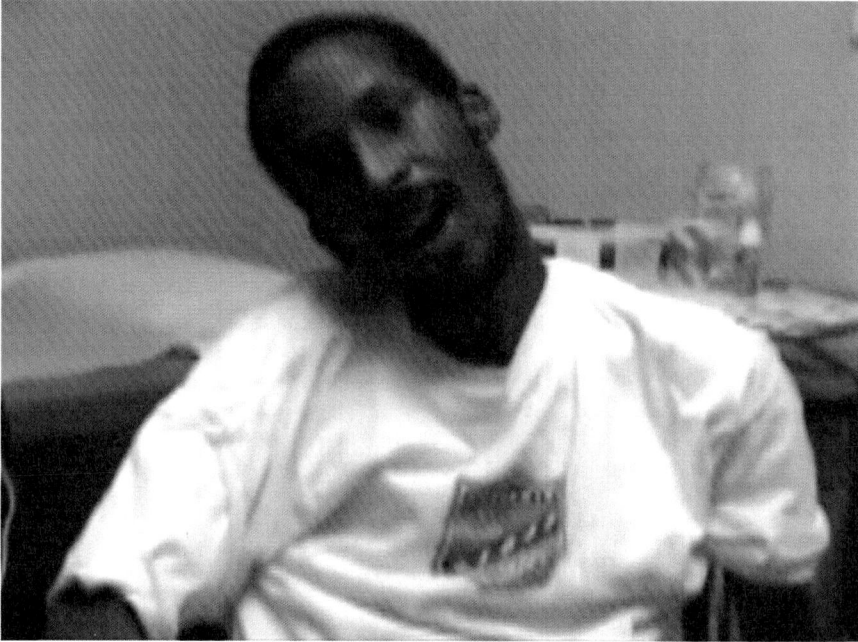

Video
There is facial masking and marked right laterocollis. He exhibits severe intention tremor together with a milder tremor at rest. Finger-nose testing is difficult due to severe tremor and ataxia. Pursuit eye movements are absent and he is unable to protrude his tongue.

References

1. Nakano KK, Dawson DM, Spence A. Machado disease. A hereditary ataxia in Portuguese emigrants to Massachusetts. Neurology. 1972;22:49–55.
2. Rosenberg RN. Mchado-Joseph disease: an autosomal dominant motor system degeneration. Mov Disord. 1992;7:193–203.
3. Kawaguchi Y, Okamoto T, Taniwaki M, et al. CAG expansions in a novel gene for Machado-Joseph disease at chromosome 14q32.1. Nat Genet. 1994;8:221–8.

Chapter 100
Spinocerebellar Ataxia-Type 6

This chapter contains a video segment which can be found at the
URL: http://www.springerimages.com/Tarsy

Background

Spinocerebellar ataxia-type 6 (SCA6) is an autosomal dominant cerebellar ataxia.
The mutation causing the disease has recently been characterized as an expanded
CAG trinucleotide repeat in the gene coding for the α_{1A}-subunit of the voltage-
dependent calcium channel. By contrast with the more common SCA2, SCA6 presents as a milder disorder, most often manifesting as a "pure" or isolated cerebellar
ataxia, accompanied by dysarthria and gaze-evoked nystagmus. Eye movements are
among the key findings in SCA6, including downbeat nystagmus, difficulty fixating
on moving objects, and diplopia but without marked functional deficits. Onset is
typically at about age 50 years but ranges widely. Noncerebellar symptoms occur
infrequently including reduced vibration and position sense, impaired upward gaze,
and spasticity late in the disease.

In SCA6, disease progresses more slowly than in other SCAs and is usually compatible with a normal life span. Late-onset symptoms may obscure the hereditary
character of ataxia if parents have died before disease onset or if gait disorders were
erroneously attributed to age. This may explain why SCA6 is found in about 10% of
patients with apparently sporadic ataxia with onset of symptoms beyond age 40.

Case

A 55-year-old woman presented with gait instability 2 years previously. Progression
was slow, but she noticed a steady decline in ambulation until she began to fall when
turning. Examination revealed a mildly wide-based gait and mild dysarthria. Finger-
nose testing was mildly impaired, and rapid alternating movements were ataxic
bilaterally.

References

1. Schols L, Kruger R, Amoiridis G, et al. Spinocerebellar ataxia type 6: genotype and phenotype
   in German kindreds. J Neurol Neurosurg Psychiatry. 1998;64:67–73.
2. Kordasiewicz HB, Gomez CM. Molecular pathogenesis of spinocerebellar ataxia type 6.
   Neurotherapeutics. 2007;4:285–94.

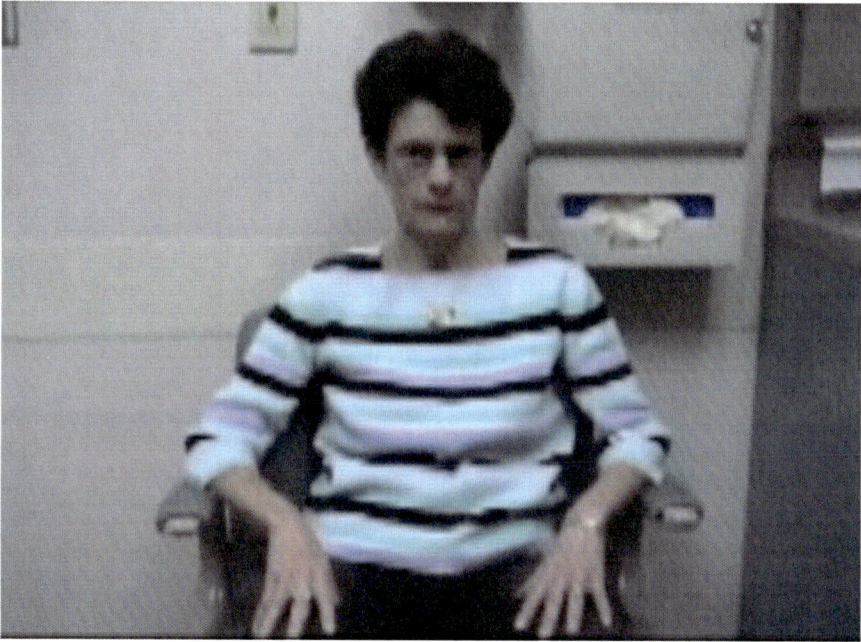

Video

The patient uses a walker because of gait ataxia. She exhibits signs of cerebellar dysfunction including a mildly wide-based gait, slow and ataxic rapid alternating movements, left-sided finger-nose ataxia, and mild dysarthria.

Chapter 101
Spinocerebellar Ataxia-Type 7

This chapter contains a video segment which can be found at the
URL: http://www.springerimages.com/Tarsy

Background

Spinocerebellar ataxia-type 7 (SCA7) is a progressive autosomal dominant neurodegenerative disorder characterized by cerebellar ataxia associated with progressive
macular dystrophy. The disease primarily affects the cerebellum and retina and is
caused by expansion of an unstable trinucleotide CAG repeat on chromosome 3 which
encodes a polyglutamine tract in the corresponding protein, ataxin-7. Pathological
alleles contain from 36 to 306 CAG repeats. The clinical hallmark of SCA7 is the
association of hereditary ataxia together with progressive visual loss caused by pigmentary macular degeneration. This association represents a distinct disease entity
originally classified as an autosomal dominant cerebellar ataxia type II by Anita
Harding. The first sign of retinal involvement is dyschromatopsia in the blue-yellow
axis or reduced central visual acuity, which can occur many years before the onset of
ataxia. It is the only SCA which may be associated with blindness. Instability of
expanded repeats is more pronounced in SCA7 than in other SCA subtypes and can
cause substantial lowering of the age of onset in successive generations so that sometimes children may become affected before their parents develop symptoms.

Case

A 44-year-old man was referred for evaluation of slowly progressive gait unsteadiness.
His initial symptom was blurred vision 9 years previously. He reported difficulty identifying colors associated with progressive loss of central vision and ability to focus.
During the past 4 years, he experienced progressive dysarthric speech. Family history
revealed that his father walked with a "funny" gait but was not neurologically evaluated. His brother had also complained of hand clumsiness for the past 2 years. He had
four children and his eldest son, now 10 years old, developed an unsteady gait at the age
of 2 and has become unable to read. His 2-year-old daughter had developmental regres-
sion and required a gastrostomy tube for feeding. Examination of the patient disclosed
visual acuity of 20/100 bilaterally associated with impaired color vision in the blue-
yellow axis. Fundoscopy revealed granular macular pigmentation interspersed with
pale areas of pigmentary atrophy (Fig. 101.1). He had mild cerebellar dysarthria. His
gait was slightly wide-based and he had difficulty with tandem gait. Examination of his
son revealed visual acuity limited to counting fingers. Ophthalmoplegia was present in
all directions of gaze associated with very slow saccades. Dysarthria was prominent.

R. Bhidayasiri, D. Tarsy, *Movement Disorders: A Video Atlas*, Current Clinical Neurology,   218
DOI 10.1007/978-1-60327-426-5_101, © Springer Science+Business Media New York 2012

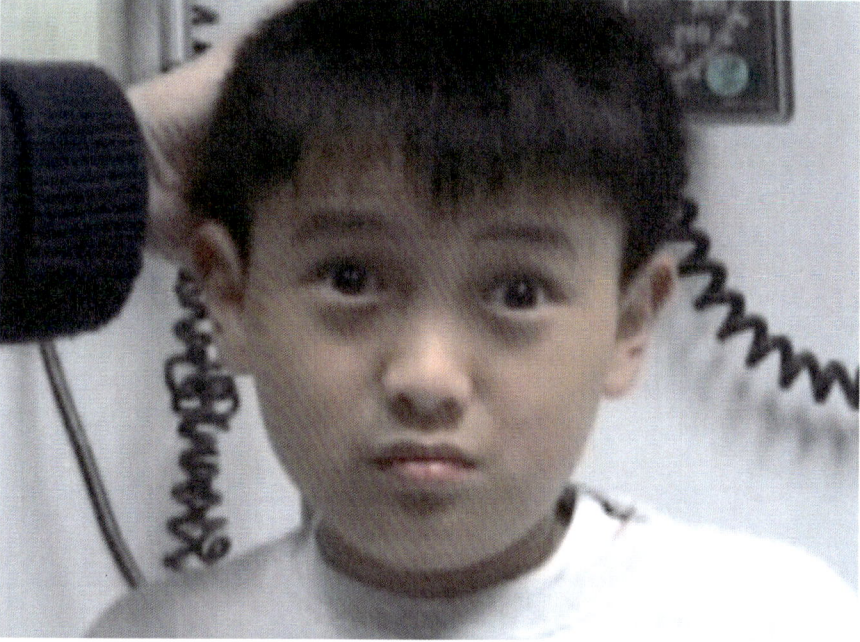

Video

Clip 1: Examination of the index patient shows mild cerebellar dysfunction with slight finger-nose ataxia, normal rapid alternating movements, a mildly wide-based gait, and difficulty with tandem gait. *Clip 2*: Examination of the index patient's nearly blind son shows ophthalmoplegia in all directions of gaze with difficulty generating saccadic and pursuit eye movements. Rapid alternating hand movements are slow, and severe finger-nose ataxia is present which appears at least in part due to poor vision. There was severe truncal and gait ataxia requiring assistance with walking.

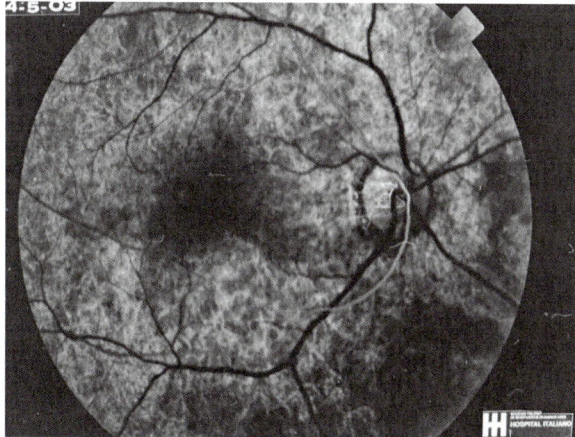

Fig. 101.1 Fundus photograph showed granular retinal epithelial changes and optic disc pallor.

References

1. McLaughlin ME, Dryja TP. Ocular findings in spinocerebellar ataxia type 7. Arch Ophthalmol. 2002;120:655–9.
2. Harding AE. The clinical features and classification of the late onset autosomal dominant cerebellar ataxias: a study of 11 families, including descendants of the 'the Drew family of Walworth'. Brain. 1982;105:1–28.
3. Enevoldson TP, Sanders MD, Harding AE. Autosomal dominant cerebellar ataxia with pigmentary macular dystrophy. A clinical and genetic study of eight families. Brain. 1994;117:445–60.

Chapter 102
Spinocerebellar Ataxia-Type 17

This chapter contains a video segment which can be found at the
URL: http://www.springerimages.com/Tarsy

Background

Spinocerebellar ataxia-type 17 (SCA17) is an autosomal dominant cerebellar ataxia
with a complex and variable phenotype characterized by ataxia, dementia, chorea,
dystonia, and parkinsonism. Affected patients typically present in early or middle
adulthood (mean age 33 years) with progressive gait and limb ataxia which is usually accompanied by dementia, psychiatric symptoms, and variable extrapyramidal
features. Additional symptoms and signs such as hyperreflexia, saccadic slowing,
akinesia, mutism, and seizures may develop, reflecting widespread cerebral and cerebellar involvement. The diagnosis of SCA17 relies on genetic testing to detect an
abnormal CAA/CAG repeat expansion in TATA-binding protein (*TBP*), the only
gene abnormality known to be associated with SCA17. Affected individuals usually
have more than 42 repeats. Some patients have only psychiatric symptoms and others present with choreiform movements similar to Huntington's disease. Brain MRI
shows variable atrophy of the cerebrum, brainstem, and cerebellum. Neuropathologic
examination shows atrophy of the striatum which is greater in the caudate nucleus.
Loss of cortical neurons occurs in some individuals. Although considered rare
among Caucasians, SCA17 should be considered in sporadic and familial cases of
ataxia when accompanied by psychiatric symptoms and dementia.

Case

A 15-year-old man was referred because of an unexplained gait disturbance. His
initial symptoms were staggering while running and inability to catch up with his
peers. For the past few years, he had episodes of loss of consciousness which were
attributed to epileptic seizures. Recently, he was diagnosed with depression with
mild paranoid psychosis. Examination disclosed mild gait ataxia and difficulty
with tandem gait. Mild right-sided parkinsonism was present. The diagnosis of
SCA17 was made on the basis of an abnormal CAA/CAG repeat expansion in the
TBP gene.

R. Bhidayasiri, D. Tarsy, *Movement Disorders: A Video Atlas*, Current Clinical Neurology,
DOI 10.1007/978-1-60327-426-5_102, © Springer Science+Business Media New York 2012

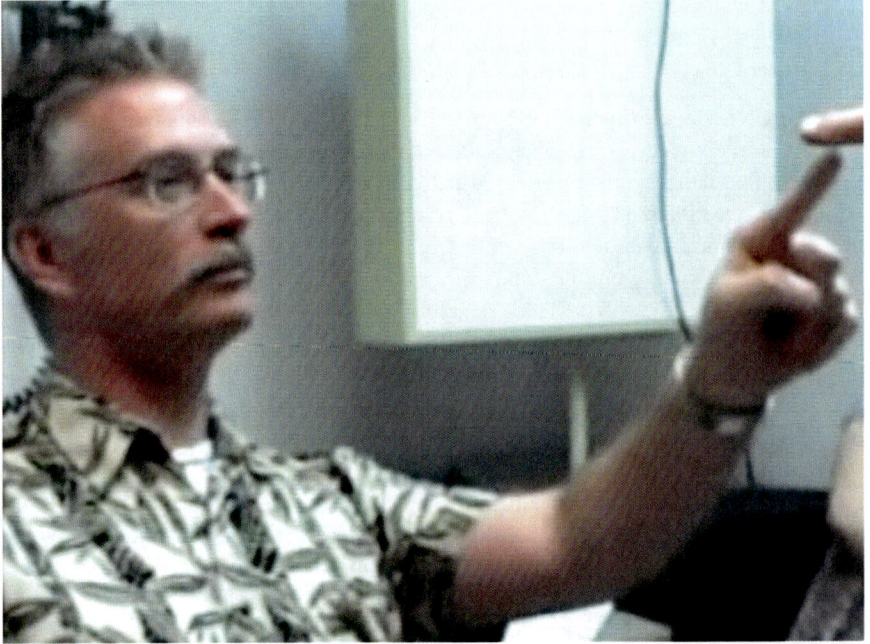

Video

Clip 1: examination exhibits only reduced left arm swing. Gait appears normal, although subjectively he finds it more difficult to perform tandem gait than 2 years previously. *Clip 2*: another patient with SCA17 shows mild finger-nose ataxia on the right side and dysarthric, scanning speech. Gait is ataxic requiring use of a walker. (Video contribution from Dr. Susan Perlman, Department of Neurology at David Geffen School of Medicine at UCLA.)

References

1. Rolfs A, Koeppen AH, Bauer I, et al. Clinical features and neuropathology of autosomal dominant spinocerebellar ataxia (SCA17). Ann Neurol. 2003;54:367–75.
2. Nakamura K, Jeong SY, Uchihara T, et al. SCA17, a novel autosomal dominant cerebellar ataxia caused by an expanded polyglutamine in TATA-binding protein. Hum Mol Genet. 2001;10:1441–8.

Chapter 103
Ataxia with Oculomotor Apraxia-Type 1

This chapter contains a video segment which can be found at the
URL: http://www.springerimages.com/Tarsy

Background

Ataxia with oculomotor apraxia-type 1 (AOA1) is an early onset ataxia with oculomotor apraxia and hypoalbuminemia. It is an autosomal recessive cerebellar ataxia
(ARCA) associated with hypoalbuminemia and hypercholesterolemia. The responsible gene *APTX*, which encodes ataprataxin, has recently been identified. In most
families, the phenotype is characterized by early onset cerebellar ataxia, oculomotor
apraxia, neuropathy, and mental retardation. The most distinctive clinical signs in
AOA1 are abnormal eye movements including gaze-evoked nystagmus (100%),
oculomotor apraxia (86%), saccadic pursuit, fixational instability, and excessive
blinking. In advanced stages, oculomotor apraxia may be masked by progressive
external ophthalmoparesis, beginning with upward vertical gaze palsy. Laboratory
findings include hypoalbuminemia and hypercholesterolemia. Elevated creatine
kinase is occasionally present. Nerve conduction velocity studies show a sensorimotor axonal neuropathy. Brain MRI shows cerebellar atrophy, mild brainstem
atrophy, and, in advanced cases, cortical atrophy. The presence of chorea, sensorimotor neuropathy, oculomotor abnormalities, biological abnormalities, and cerebellar atrophy on neuroimaging and the absence of Babinski signs can help
distinguish AOA1 from Friedreich's ataxia clinically.

Based on study of one of the largest series of patients with molecular proven
AOA1, the relative frequency of AOA1 is 5.7% in families with progressive cerebellar ataxia. AOA1 was originally described in Japan where it is considered to be the
most common cause of ARCA. It is the second most common cause of ARCA in
Portugal.

Case

An 18-year-old woman experienced gait instability associated with dysarthria and
developmental delay since childhood. Her condition gradually progressed until she
required assistance with all daily activities due to marked ataxia, dysarthria, dysphagia, and tremor. On examination, the patient exhibited marked dysarthria, titubation, postural hand tremor, hyporeflexia, and flexor plantar responses. Detailed
ocular examination revealed oculomotor apraxia, particularly in horizontal gaze.
Biochemical tests revealed hypoalbuminemia and hypercholesterolemia. Genetic
testing disclosed a mutation of the *APTX* gene.

R. Bhidayasiri, D. Tarsy, *Movement Disorders: A Video Atlas*, Current Clinical Neurology,   224
DOI 10.1007/978-1-60327-426-5_103, © Springer Science+Business Media New York 2012

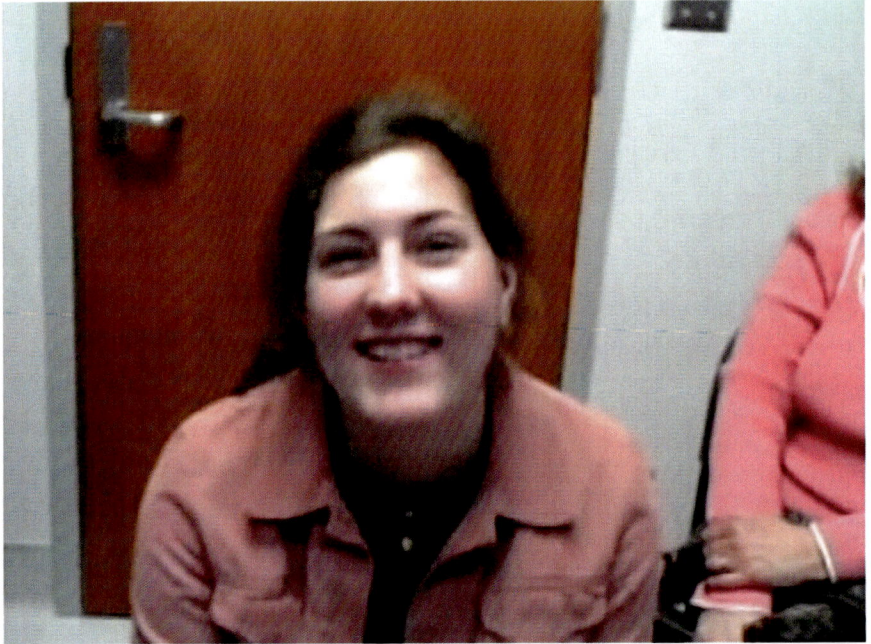

Video

Clip 1: the eye movement examination shows oculomotor apraxia in horizontal gaze. *Clip 2*: the patient has marked gait ataxia characterized by a wide-based gait. Upper extremities are also ataxic. (Video contribution from Dr. Susan Perlman, Department of Neurology at David Geffen School of Medicine at UCLA.)

References

1. Le Ber I, Moreira MC, Rivaud-Pechoux S, et al. Cerebellar ataxia with oculomotor apraxia type 1: clinical and genetic studies. Brain. 2003;126:2761–72.
2. Inoue I, Izumi K, Matawari S, et al. Congenital ocular motor apraxia and cerebellar degeneration-report of two cases. Rinsho Shinkeigaku. 1971;11:855–61.
3. Moreira MC, Barbot C, Tachi N, et al. The gene mutated in ataxia-ocular apraxia 1 encodes the new HIT/Zn-finger protein aprataxin. Nat Genet. 2001;29:189–93.

Chapter 104
Ataxia with Oculomotor Apraxia-Type 2

This chapter contains a video segment which can be found at the
URL: http://www.springerimages.com/Tarsy

Background

Ataxia with oculomotor apraxia-type 2 (AOA2) is an autosomal recessive disorder due
to mutations in the senataxin gene causing progressive cerebellar ataxia with peripheral
neuropathy, cerebellar atrophy, oculomotor apraxia, and elevated alpha-fetoprotein
(AFP) serum levels. The onset of the disease is usually between ages 12 and 20. The
increase in AFP level as well as cerebellar atrophy seems to be stable during the course
of the disease and to occur mostly at or before disease onset. The clinical phenotype is
characterized by progressive cerebellar ataxia, sensorimotor peripheral neuropathy,
oculomotor apraxia in 51% of cases, strabismus, chorea, and dystonia. Frontal executive dysfunction may be disturbed. Premature ovarian failure has been reported in some
patients. The clinical phenotype is fairly homogeneous, showing only subtle intrafamil-
ial variability. Progression is slow and most patients are wheelchair-bound 10 years
after onset. In addition to an elevated AFP level, increased serum creatine kinase, cho-
lesterol, IgG, IgA, and hypoalbuminemia sometimes occur.

Relative frequency of AOA2 is 8% of non-Friedreich's autosomal recessive cerebellar ataxias which is more frequent than ataxic-telangiectasia (AT) and AOA1.
The probability for a non-Friedreich's ataxia, non-AT ataxic patient to be affected
with AOA2 with AFP level ≥7 μg/l is 46%. The normal level of AFP ranges from
0.5 to 17.2 μg/l. Therefore, selection of patients with an AFP level above 7 μg/l for
senataxin gene sequencing is a good strategy for AOA2 diagnosis.

Case

A 23-year-old man presented with a 5 year history of progressive gait instability and
slurred speech. Examination revealed marked dysarthria, cerebellar ataxia in all
extremities, absent reflexes in both legs, and oculomotor apraxia in horizontal gaze.
AFP level was elevated at 31 μg/l. The diagnosis of AOA2 was confirmed by the
presence of a mutation in the senataxin gene.

R. Bhidayasiri, D. Tarsy, *Movement Disorders: A Video Atlas*, Current Clinical Neurology,   226
DOI 10.1007/978-1-60327-426-5_104, © Springer Science+Business Media New York 2012

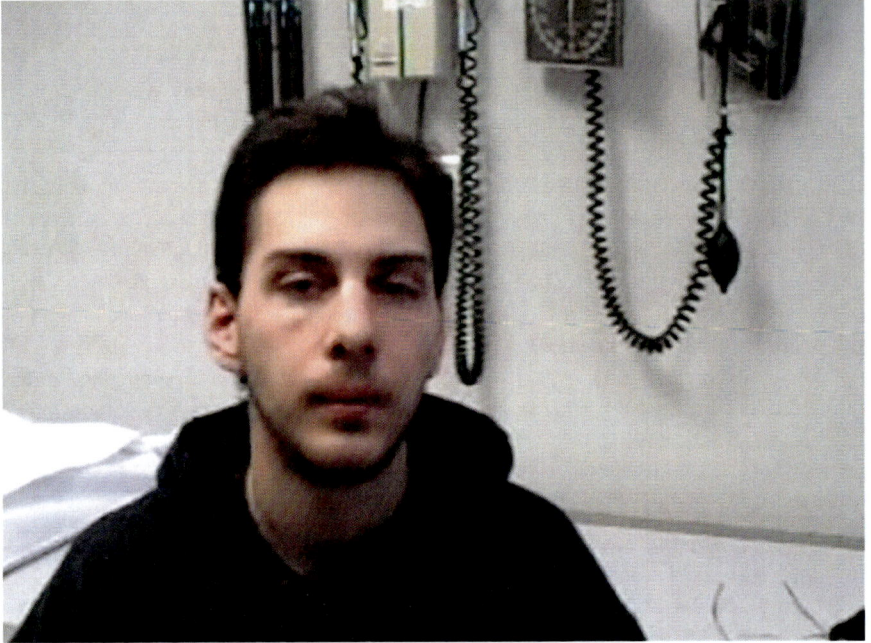

Video

Clip 1: the patient exhibits oculomotor apraxia with inability to generate saccadic eye movements with or without a visual target. Eye movements are intact with oculocephalic maneuvers. Bilateral ataxia with finger-nose movements is also present. *Clip 2*: the same patient displays gait ataxia. (Video contribution from Dr. Susan Perlman, Department of Neurology at David Geffen School of Medicine at UCLA.)

References

1. Anheim M, Monga B, Fleury M, et al. Ataxia with oculomotor apraxia type 2: clinical, biological, and genotype/phenotype correlation study of a cohort of 90 patients. Brain. 2009;132:2688–98.
2. Le Ber I, Bouslam N, Rivaud-Pechoux S, et al. Frequency and phenotypic spectrum of ataxia with oculomotor apraxia 2: a clinical and genetic study in 18 patients. Brain. 2004;127:759–67.
3. Criscuolo C, Chessa L, Di Giandomenico S, et al. Ataxia with oculomotor apraxia type 2: a clinical, pathologic, and genetic study. Neurology. 2006;66:1207–10.

Chapter 105
Friedreich's Ataxia

This chapter contains a video segment which can be found at the
URL: http://www.springerimages.com/Tarsy

Background

Friedreich's ataxia (FRDA) is the most common of the autosomal recessive cerebellar ataxias. According to the Harding's criteria, FRDA begins before the end of puberty or at least before the age of 25. The FRDA gene encodes frataxin, a protein which is involved in mitochondrial iron regulation. The phenotypic spectrum has appeared to widen since the identification of mutations in the FRDA gene. Notable atypical features include late-onset forms of FRDA and individuals with preserved tendon reflexes. Almost all patients are homozygous for a GAA expansion which occurs at the intron 1 of the FRDA gene. Normal individuals have up to 40 GAA repeats, but this number may vary from 70 to over 1,700 repeats. The presence of biallelic expansion confirms the diagnosis. The size of expanded repeats on GAA1 is inversely related to age at onset and disease severity in FRDA, but GAA2 size is a poor predictor of clinical variation.

Gait instability is nearly always the initial manifestation of FRDA and disease progression is usually relentless, resulting in most patients becoming wheelchair-bound within 10–15 years of disease onset. Patients with late-onset FRDA tend to have a milder and more slowly evolving course which is associated with a shorter GAA expansion. Other features of FRDA include dysarthria, reduced vibration and proprioceptive sense, absence of deep tendon reflexes, extensor plantar responses, instability of ocular fixation, pes cavus, and scoliosis. Systemic manifestations include hypertrophic cardiomyopathy, cardiac conduction defects, and diabetes mellitus.

Case

A 17-year-old woman presented with gait instability which had become progressively worse during the previous 2 years. A maternal aunt was affected with a similar condition. Examination revealed a wide-based gait and need for assistance with ambulation. Speech was mildly dysarthric. Tendon reflexes were absent and plantar responses were extensor. Vibration and joint position sense were severely diminished in the lower limbs. She was not diabetic, and transthoracic echocardiography showed no evidence for cardiomyopathy.

R. Bhidayasiri, D. Tarsy, *Movement Disorders: A Video Atlas*, Current Clinical Neurology,
DOI 10.1007/978-1-60327-426-5_105, © Springer Science+Business Media New York 2012

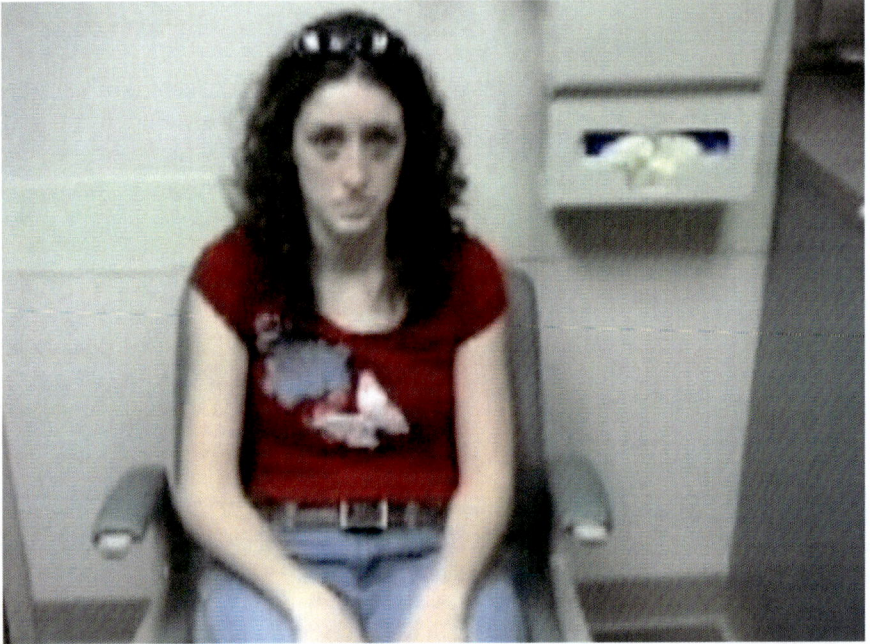

Video

The patient exhibits a characteristic wide-based gait with need for assistance. There is a bilateral foot drop due to coexisting peripheral motor neuropathy. Speech is dysarthric. Ocular examination showed unsustained gaze-evoked horizontal nystagmus. Finger-nose testing is ataxic bilaterally. Pes cavus is present.

References

1. Pandolfo M. Friedreich's Ataxia. Arch Neurol. 2008;65:1296–303.
2. Bhidayasiri R, Perlman SL, Pulse SM, Geschwind DH. Late-onset Friedreich ataxia: phenotypic analysis, magnetic resonance imaging findings, and review of the literature. Arch Neurol. 2005;62:1865–9.
3. Fogel BL, Perlman S. Clinical features and molecular genetics of autosomal recessive ataxias. Lancet Neurol. 2007;6:245–57.

Chapter 106
Multiple System Atrophy with Cerebellar Ataxia

This chapter contains a video segment which can be found at the
URL: http://www.springerimages.com/Tarsy

Background

Multiple system atrophy with predominant cerebellar ataxia (MSA-C) is a sporadic
disorder which usually presents as a midline cerebellar disorder which progresses
more rapidly than other late-onset sporadic ataxias. The patient typically becomes
wheelchair-dependent within 5 years of onset. Diagnostic criteria for probable
MSA-C include a sporadic, progressive adult-onset cerebellar syndrome together
with additional features of parkinsonism, Babinski signs, and laryngeal stridor.
Interestingly, cerebellar ataxia often improves as signs of parkinsonism emerge later
in the disease. A recent consensus statement emphasizes neuroimaging features
including atrophy of the putamen, middle cerebellar peduncle, or pons; FDG-PET
hypometabolism in the putamen; and presynaptic nigrostriatal dopaminergic dener-
vation with SPECT or PET imaging. However, clinicians evaluating patients with
progressive ataxia should consider a range of differential diagnostic possibilities
because there are numerous disorders which produce an adult-onset, progressive
cerebellar ataxia. Dominantly inherited spinocerebellar ataxias (SCAs) may also
cause an apparently sporadic disorder since there is a 15–20% chance of a mutation
in one of several polyglutamine SCAs, notably SCA1, 2, 3, 6, and 7. Fragile
X-associated tremor/ataxia syndrome is a neurodegenerative disorder with core features of action tremor and ataxia of gait. A family history of a similar disorder
makes the diagnosis of MSA-C unlikely, and one of the SCAs should be considered.
Dementia also makes the diagnosis of MSA-C unlikely.

Case

A 52-year-old woman was referred to an emergency room with sudden onset of
inspiratory stridor requiring emergency tracheostomy. Further investigation revealed
abductor laryngeal paresis. Examination showed that she was slow with facial masking. Her gait was unsteady and she was unable to perform tandem gait. Rapid finger
tapping was mildly bradykinetic bilaterally. There was no family history of ataxia.

R. Bhidayasiri, D. Tarsy, *Movement Disorders: A Video Atlas*, Current Clinical Neurology,
DOI 10.1007/978-1-60327-426-5_106, © Springer Science+Business Media New York 2012

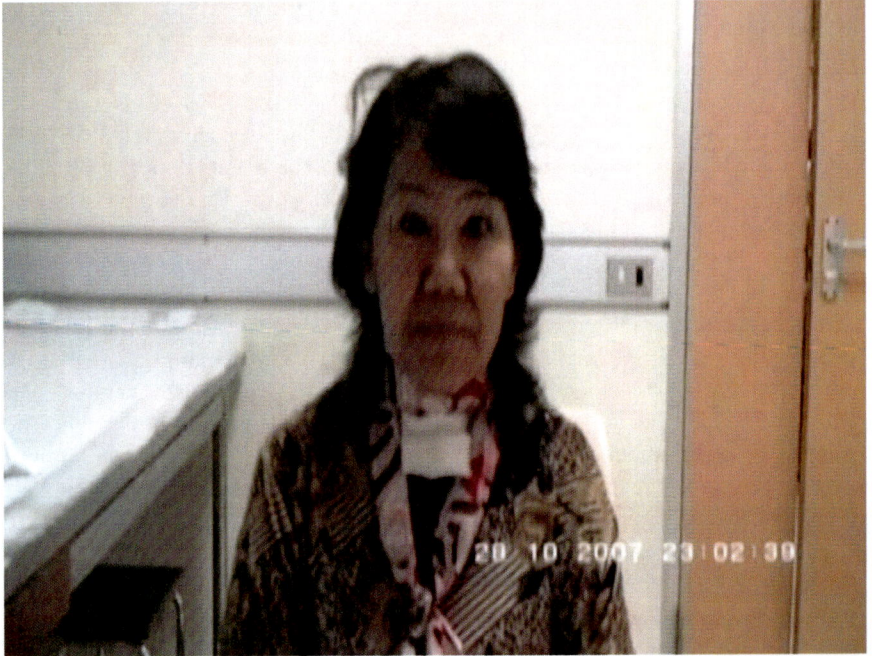

Video

Clip 1: the patient shows evidence of mild facial masking and parkinsonism, but the cerebellar features are more prominent including gait ataxia and inability to perform tandem gait. *Clip 2*: at follow-up examination 18 months later, facial masking has become more prominent, and the upper extremities and gait have become more ataxic. She now requires assistance to walk for a few steps and she has become wheelchair-dependent.

References

1. Silber MH, Levine S. Stridor and death in multiple system atrophy. Mov Disord. 2000;15:699–704.
2. Bhidayasiri R, Ling H. Multiple system atrophy. Neurologist. 2008;14:224–37.
3. Gilman S, Wenning GK, Low PA, et al. Second consensus statement on the diagnosis of multiple system atrophy. Neurology. 2008;71:670–6.

Part VII
Tic Disorders

Chapter 107
Motor Tic Disorder

This chapter contains a video segment which can be found at the
URL: http://www.springerimages.com/Tarsy

Background

Tics are defined as brief, intermittent, nonrhythmic, unpredictable, purposeless movements (motor tics) or sounds (phonic or vocal tics). They are frequently associated with a subjective urge to carry out the tic. Voluntary suppression results in psychic tension and anxiety which are relieved with the "release" created by executing the movements or sounds. The diagnosis of Tourette syndrome requires the presence of both motor and vocal or verbal tics (see Chap. 109).

Tics are classified as simple or complex. Simple motor tics are focal movements involving one group of muscles such as eye blinking, tongue protrusion, facial grimacing, shoulder shrugging, and head turning. Complex motor tics are coordinated or sequential patterns of movements that may resemble normal motor tasks or gestures. Examples include head shaking, arm twisting, obscene gestures such as "giving the finger" (copropraxia), and imitating gestures of others (echopraxia). Motor tics can also be classified according to the speed of movement. When they are brief, sudden, or jerk-like, they are called clonic tics. Motor tics that involve twisting movements and abnormal postures are called dystonic tics. Those which produce sustained prolonged movements and postures are called tonic tics.

Case

The family of a 15-year-old boy noticed that he had intermittent facial movements. Examination showed intermittent episodes of eye blinking and frowning. Although he was able to suppress the movements for a brief period, the effect was only temporary and created internal sensations of tension and discomfort. He experienced no vocal tics. It was noted that his father had frequent head turning movements.

References

1. Jankovic J. Tourette's syndrome: phenomenology and classification of tics. Neurol Clin. 1997;15:267–75.
2. Evidente VG. Is it a tic or Tourette's? Clues for differentiating simple from more complex tic disorders. Postgrad Med. 2000;108:175–82.

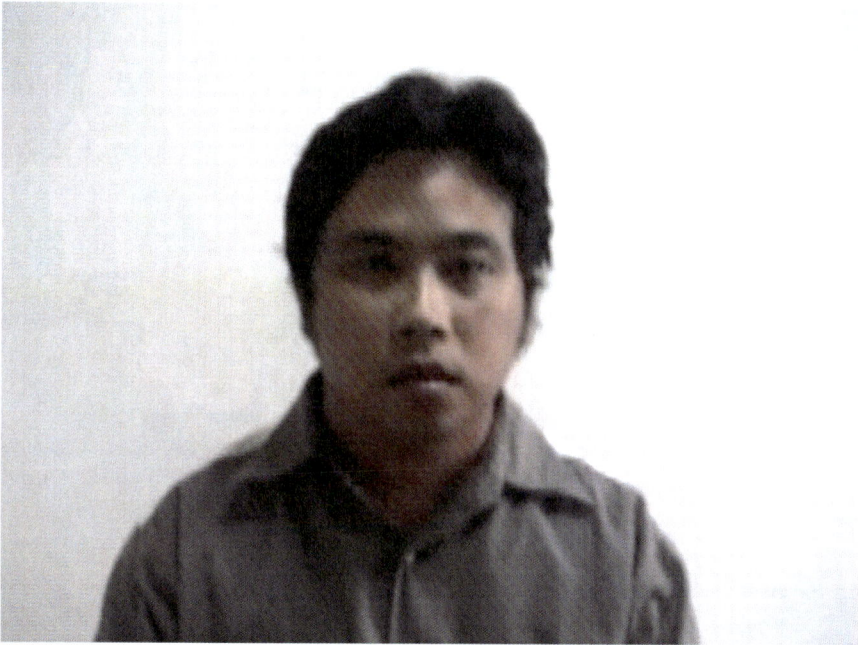

Video

Clip 1: the patient exhibits increased eye blinking frequency and repetitive frowning which increase while carrying out rapid movements. *Clip 2*: another 14-year-old boy displays complex motor tics with sequential large amplitude rotational and hyperextension head movements, arm twisting, shoulder shrugging, and jumping and twisting leg movements. He reports that the movements are painful, but that he is unable to voluntarily stop them. He lacks vocal tics.

Chapter 108
Adult Onset Tic Disorder

This chapter contains a video segment which can be found at the
URL: http://www.springerimages.com/Tarsy

Background

According to the DSM-IV-TR criteria, the diagnosis of Tourette syndrome (TS)
includes onset before the age of 18 years. However, the symptoms of TS may persist
into adulthood, and rarely a major tic disorder may begin for the first time in adults.
Compared to childhood-onset TS, adult patients with severe tic disorders have
significantly more facial and truncal tics, and there is an association with substance
abuse and mood disorders. They have fewer phonic tics and a lower incidence of
attention deficit-hyperactivity disorder. However, most of the time, severe tic disorders in adults probably represent a reappearance or exacerbation of childhood-onset
TS. In adults, other underlying causes of "tourettism" have been reported including
postencephalitic syndrome, carbon monoxide poisoning, trauma, drug intoxica-
tions, and neurodegenerative disorders. Patients with adult-onset tics more often
have severe symptoms, greater social morbidity, potential triggering events, and
increased sensitivity to and poorer responses to treatment with neuroleptic drugs.

Case

A 52-year-old man was referred because of recent worsening of tics consisting of
violent head shaking and head banging. He stated the symptoms began 10 years
previously but had recently become more severe which he attributed to posttraumatic stress disorder. He denied any premonitory urge. Examination revealed a
cluster of violent head shaking behaviors which he could not suppress. There was
no vocalization. Neurologic examination and neuroimaging were normal.

References

1. Jankovic J, Gelineau-Kattner R, Davidson A. Tourette's Syndrome in adults. Mov Disord.
   2010;25:2171–5.
2. Eapen V, Less AJ, Lakke JP, et al. Adult-onset tic disorders. Mov Disord. 2002;17:735–40.

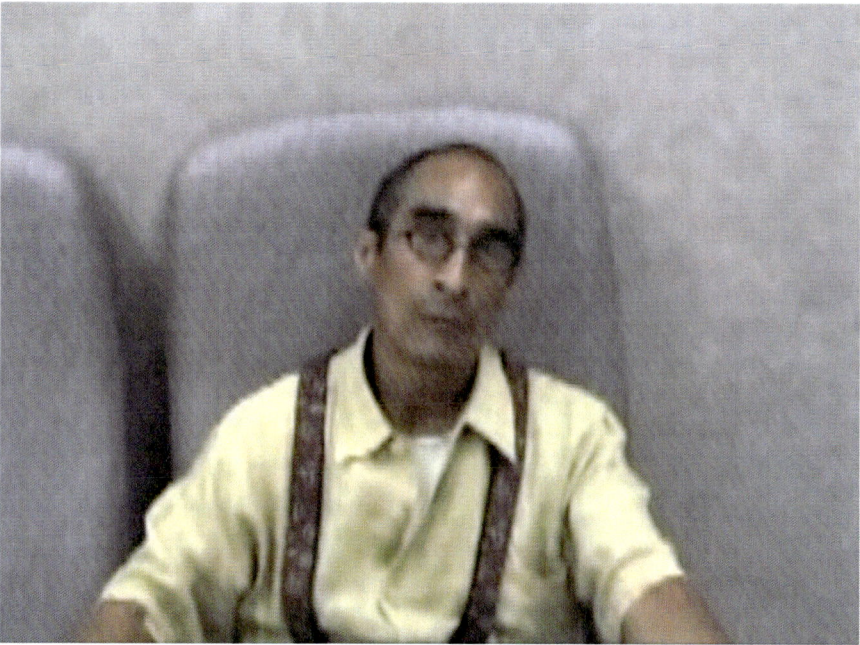

Video
The patient exhibits repetitive stereotypic movements consisting of large amplitude head shaking to one side. His left shoulder is elevated and there is a mild left laterocollis. The tics appear to subside while speaking.

Chapter 109
Tourette's Syndrome: Complex Tics

This chapter contains a video segment which can be found at the
URL: http://www.springerimages.com/Tarsy

Background

Tourette syndrome (TS) is a childhood-onset disorder characterized by chronic motor
and vocal tics which persist for more than 1 year. It is estimated that TS affects about
1% of children. Risk factors include male gender, family history of tics, obsessive-
compulsive disorder (OCD), and attention deficit-hyperactivity disorder (ADHD).
Transient tic disorders in childhood are much more common than TS. Twenty percent of children, boys more commonly than girls, have motor tics which disappear as
they get older. According to DSM-IV, the standard diagnostic criteria for TS consist
of (1) presence of multiple motor tics and one or more vocal tics, (2) tics occurring
many times daily for more than 3 consecutive months, (3) onset younger than 18 years
of age, and (4) a tic disorder not due to substance abuse or another underlying diagnosis. Vocal or phonic tics may include inarticulate noises such as throat clearing,
sniffing, coughing as well as use of words or parts of words. Sudden, obscene utter-
ances (coprolalia) occur in less than 50% of individuals with TS.

TS is considered to be a neuropsychiatric spectrum disorder which is commonly
associated with features of OCD or ADHD. Other associated behavioral disorders
sometimes include rage attacks, depression, bipolar disorder, impulse-control disorder,
self-injurious behavior, and anxiety. Tics typically wax and wane in severity over time.
As children grow into adolescence and adulthood, tics resolve in about one-third of
cases and become less severe in another third. In the remainder of cases, TS persists
lifelong without change. In many cases, tics may be mild and not disabling and education about the disorder and supportive counseling provide sufficient management.
Cognitive behavioral therapy, particularly habit-reversal treatment, is sometimes helpful
in suppressing tics. Medications are reserved for more severe cases. These include neuroleptic drugs for which the FDA has approved haloperidol and pimozide. Risperidone
may also be effective. Tetrabenazine is also helpful and does not carry the risk of causing
tardive dyskinesia. Milder cases may be successfully treated with clonazepam, cloni-
dine, or guanfacine. Thalamic and pallidal deep brain stimulations have also been used
with some success in severe cases which are unresponsive to medications.

Case

An 18-year-old man who had been diagnosed with TS 3 years previously presented
for treatment at an outpatient clinic. Symptoms were initially mild and did not

R. Bhidayasiri, D. Tarsy, *Movement Disorders: A Video Atlas*, Current Clinical Neurology,
DOI 10.1007/978-1-60327-426-5_109, © Springer Science+Business Media New York 2012

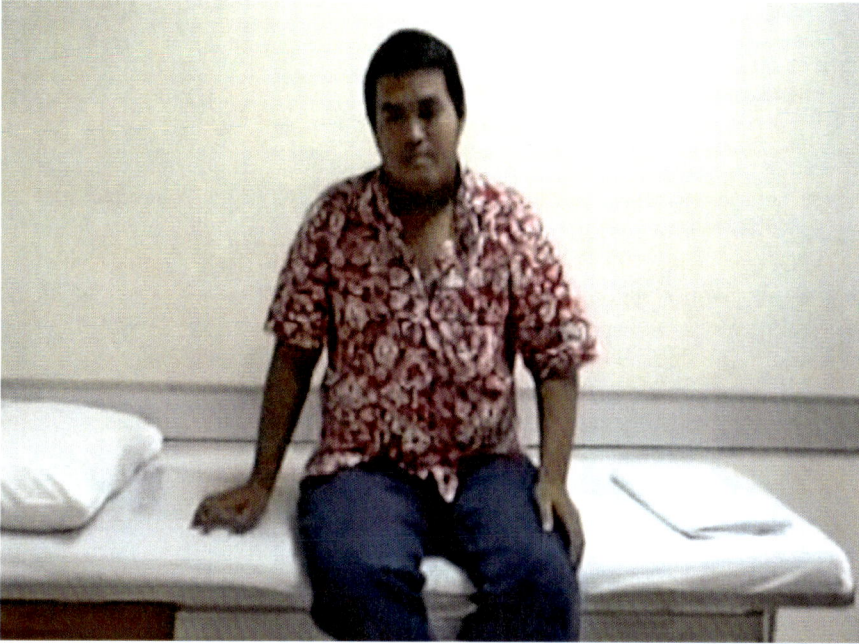

Video

The patient exhibits a series of complex motor tics consisting of sequential head shaking and turning, arm shaking and leg kicking, together with grunting and humming noises and repeating over and over again the last syllable of a word (palilalia). Walking is associated with appearance of other complex tics in all four extremities.

require pharmacologic suppression. However, during a 3-month period, tic intensity increased to include complex motor and vocal tics consisting of inarticulate noises and partial words. The tics occurred several times daily and interfered with studies and school performance.

References

1. Kurlan R. Tourette's syndrome. N Eng J Med. 2010;363:2332–8.
2. Cath D, Hedderly T, Ludolph AG, et al. European clinical guidelines for Tourette syndrome and other tic disorders part 1: assessment. Eur Child Adolesc Psychiatry. 2011;20:155–71.
3. Porta M, Brambilla A, Cavanna AE, et al. Thalamic deep brain stimulation for treatment-refractory Tourette syndrome. Neurology. 2009;73:1375–80.

Chapter 110
Tourette's Syndrome: Malignant Dystonic Tics

This chapter contains a video segment which can be found at the
URL: http://www.springerimages.com/Tarsy

Background

Tourette syndrome (TS) refers to a childhood-onset disorder with motor and phonic
tics sometimes associated with behavioral abnormalities which commonly include
obsessive-compulsive disorder (OCD) and attention deficit-hyperactivity disorder
(ADHD) (see Chap. 109). Most individuals with TS cases are only mildly affected
and do not require pharmacologic intervention. However, at the other end of the
spectrum, TS may be very severe, and its comorbid behavioral symptoms can cause
potentially life-threatening outcomes due to severe tics, extreme rage attacks,
depression with suicidal ideation, and disabling self-injurious behavior (see Chap.
111). Severe cases of this type are referred to as "malignant TS" and represent
approximately 5% of patients with TS.

Malignant TS is associated with severe motor symptoms and the presence of two
or more behavioral abnormalities. Compared with other patients with TS, these individuals are more likely to have an obsessive compulsive personality, complex phonic
tics, coprolalia, copropraxia, self-injurious behavior, mood disorders, suicidal ideation, and a poor response to medications. Obsessive-compulsive disorder appears to
play an important role in malignant TS. Although rare, recognition of this subgroup
of TS patients is important for early intervention with the hope that it will prevent or
delay life-threatening complications. Thalamic and pallidal deep brain stimulation
may be the only available therapeutic option in such cases and has been successful.

Case

A 16-year-old man had a history of complex motor tics including head shaking and
shoulder shrugging since age 14. He had difficulty paying attention in school.
Obsessive-compulsive behaviors such as recurrent thoughts and checking emerged
in his early teens. He quit school 2 years previously because of symptoms of ADHD.
During the previous year, he developed complex motor tics including an irresistible
urge to forcefully hyperextend his neck until he would hear a "clicking sound" at
extreme hyperextension. If he did not hear or feel the "clicking" in his neck, he
would repeat the posture until he was able to achieve the "right" feeling. He tried to
resist the urge but this led to inner feelings of discomfort leading to an even stronger
compulsion to perform the maneuver. During the previous few months, he developed neck pain, numbness in both legs, and difficulty in walking. Despite these new

R. Bhidayasiri, D. Tarsy, *Movement Disorders: A Video Atlas*, Current Clinical Neurology,   240
DOI 10.1007/978-1-60327-426-5_110, © Springer Science+Business Media New York 2012

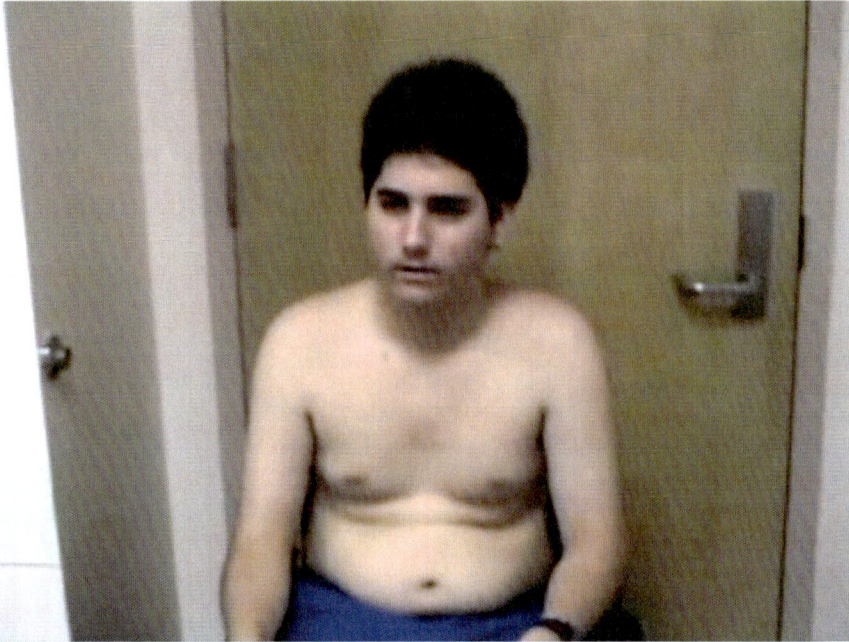

Video
The patient is sitting in a wheelchair. While speaking, he reports feeling that an inner tension is building up so that he needs to relieve the tension by forcefully hyperextending his neck until he hears or feels the "clicking" sensation. Gait is abnormal due to myelopathy.

symptoms, he continued to perform the maneuver to the point that neck pain became intense and he became unable to walk. Cervical spine MRI showed disk herniation at C5/6 and C6/7 with significant cord compression.

References

1. Cheung M-Y, Shahed J, Jankovic J. Malignant Tourette syndrome. Mov Disord. 2007;12:1743–50.
2. Krauss JK, Jankovic J. Severe motor tics causing cervical myelopathy in Tourette's syndrome. Mov Disord. 1996;11:563–6.
3. Dobbs M, Berger JR. Cervical myelopathy secondary to violent tics in Tourette's syndrome. Neurology. 2003;60:1862–3.

Chapter 111
Tourette's Syndrome: Self-Injurious Behavior

This chapter contains a video segment which can be found at the
URL: http://www.springerimages.com/Tarsy

Background

Self-injurious behavior (SIB) refers to deliberate, non-accidental, repetitive infliction
of self-harm without suicidal intent. Although SIB is present in approximately 4%
of general psychiatric patients, it occurs in up to 60% of patients with Tourette syndrome (TS). A variety of minor and major forms of SIB have been reported, including compulsive skin picking, lip biting, filing the teeth, head banging, self hitting,
eye damage from self poking, self cutting, and even castration.

SIB is correlated with the severity of tic symptoms and with high levels of obses-
siveness and hostility. Individuals with TS plus at least one other psychiatric morbidity have a fourfold increased risk of SIB. There is also a positive linear relationship
between the number of psychiatric comorbidities and the presence of SIB. It is currently unclear if SIB in TS represents a compulsion, problems with impulse regulation, or both. However, prompt recognition and treatment of SIB in TS is important
in order to prevent severe or permanent injuries in these patients.

Case

A 14-year-old boy with a 2-year history of TS presented with intermittent episodes
of uncontrollable self-hitting. His usual TS symptoms included head shaking, arm
twisting, and leg kicking, which were partially controlled with haloperidol. He
recently began to display episodes in which he would injure himself by hitting his
own body or surrounding objects. These episodes could not be suppressed as he felt
an intense urge to relieve an inner tension with this behavior. More recently, he hit
walls and other objects at home leading to numerous cuts and bruises. Some of these
injuries required emergency room visits for treatment.

References

1. Matthews CA, Waller J, Glidden DV, et al. Self injurious behaviour in Tourette syndrome: correlates with impulsivity and impulse control. J Neurol Neurosurg Psychiatry. 2004;75:1149–55.
2. Robertson MM, Trimble MR, Lees AJ. Self-injurious behavior and the Gilles de la Tourtte
syndrome: A clinical study and review of the literature. Psychol Med. 1989;19:611–25.

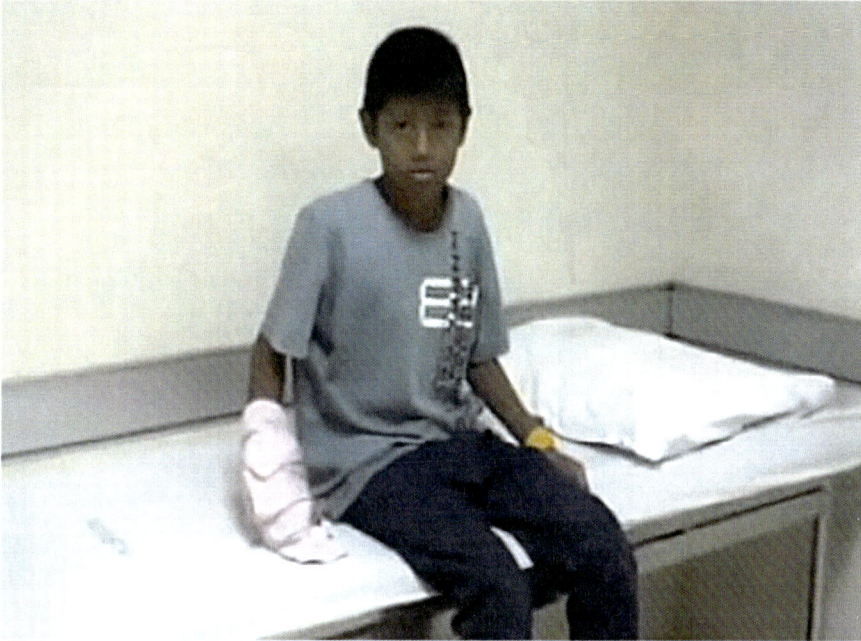

Video
The patient has a towel wrapped around his hand in order to prevent injury. He exhibits violent episodes of hitting a wall and occasionally hitting himself. Some of the episodes are associated with violent shouting or screaming.

Index

Printed by Publishers' Graphics LLC